Effective Clinical Supervision:
The role of reflection

Other titles in the series:

- *Reflection: Principles and practice for healthcare professionals* by Tony Ghaye and Sue Lillyman

- *Empowerment Through Reflection: The narratives of healthcare professionals* edited by Tony Ghaye, Dave Gillespie and Sue Lillyman

- *Caring Moments: The discourse of reflective practice* edited by Tony Ghaye and Sue Lillyman

- *The Reflective Mentor* by Sue Lillyman and Tony Ghaye

Effective Clinical Supervision:
The role of reflection

edited by

Tony Ghaye and Sue Lillyman

Quay Books

Mark Allen Publishing Ltd

Quay Books Division, Mark Allen Publishing Group
Jesses Farm, Snow Hill, Dinton, Wiltshire, SP3 5HN

British Library Cataloguing-in-Publication Data
A catalogue record is available for this book

© Mark Allen Publishing Ltd 2000
ISBN 1 85642 125 2

Printed in the UK by The Cromwell Press, Trowbridge, Wiltshire

Contents

Contributors   vii

Acknowledgements   xiii

Introduction. Colleague-centred care: The re-framing of clinical supervision   xv
Tony Ghaye

1   Sowing the seeds of clinical supervision   1
Helen Roden

2   Challenging values in clinical supervision through reflective conversations   19
David Eltringham, Penny Gill-Cripps and Margaret Lawless

3   Some reflections on the implementation of clinical supervision   45
Gail Parsons

4   The role of reflection in nurturing creative clinical conversations   55
Tony Ghaye

5   Connecting reflective practice with clinical supervision   73
Dawn Pattison, Dorothy Parsons and Clare Weatherhead

6   An alternative training approach in clinical supervision   93
John Cutcliffe

Index   115

Contributors

John Cutliffe RMN, RGN, BSc(Hons)
Senior Lecturer in Mental Health

I have been nursing since 1987. I trained first as a mental health nurse, then a general nurse and completed my BSc (Hons) in Nursing in 1990. My clinical background includes work within liaison psychiatry, care of the older person and predominantly of individuals with severe and enduring mental illness. I took up research in 1994 and this developed into a secondment to Nottingham University. I have produced 45 publications covering a wide range of topics but focusing on hope, clinical supervision, counselling, qualitative methodologies and the nature of mental health nursing. My interest in clinical supervision has been consistent throughout my career as a recipient, provider, teacher and/or researcher.

David Eltringham RGN, DNSc, BA Ed (Hons) Reflective Practice
Home Manager, Ravenstone Nursing and Residential Home, Droitwich

I am a registered general nurse with eleven years' experience in the health service working in a range of organisations and medical specialities. I became involved in clinical supervision in 1996 and, as a result, developed a strong interest in reflective practice. I believe that clinical supervision is an important part of professional development which encourages practitioners to challenge their values and beliefs in a safe and structured way. I also believe that this process will contribute significantly to clinical governance and professional self-regulation agendas. In addition, I believe that all of the registered nurses in my team should be able to access clinical supervision and I am actively involved in preparing clinical supervisors to practise, as well as supervising and being supervised themselves.

Tony Ghaye Cert Ed, B Ed (Hons), MA (Ed) PhD
Professor of Education and Director of the Policy into Practice Research Centre, University College, Worcester

In my working life I have been fortunate in being able to work with and learn from a very wide range of professionals, including nurses, midwives, health visitors, GPs, social workers, police and probation officers, therapists of various kinds, osteopaths and school teachers. I have also experienced the privilege and challenge of working with individuals and communities in the Third World and in emerging nations in North Africa and the Middle East. All this experience has energised my commitment to inter-professional learning and multi-disciplinary working to help to improve what we do with and for others. I see reflective practice and action research as a central part of my work on quality of life issues. I have just completed the largest survey of its kind undertaken in the UK into young people's attitudes towards, and behaviours in relation to, illicit drugs and alcohol. This contributed to improvements in service policy and practice. I am the founder and editor-in-chief of the multi-professional international Carfax journal, 'Reflective Practice'.

Penny Gill-Cripps RGN, City and Guilds Teaching Cert, Cert in Counselling, Dip in Management, BA Ed (Hons) Reflective Practice
Practice Development Nurse

I qualified as a registered nurse in 1978 at the Queen Elizabeth School of Nursing in Birmingham. In the last twenty years I have worked in accident and emergency, gastro-enterology and urology, and spent a year as a GP practice nurse. My passion for teaching began early in my career when I studied to be a teacher in 1990 and joined New College, Redditch where I taught psychology and health studies to pre-nursing students for four years. My present post of practice development nurse combines the two loves of my life — nursing practice and teaching, and it was this post that initiated my passion for clinical supervision. The role of practice development nurse gives me an opportunity to be involved in many aspects of care including clinical supervision, research, reflective practice, management and care of patients whilst also supporting my colleagues.

Margaret Lawless RGN, Dip SN, BA Ed (Hons) Reflective Practice
Nurse Manager — Nursing Home

Having completed traditional nurse training as a mature student, I qualified as a staff nurse in 1992. I am committed to lifelong learning and completed the Diploma in Professional Nurse Studies at the University of Wolverhampton in 1995 and, in 1997, commenced a BA Ed (Hons) in Reflective Practice at University College, Worcester. My career pathway has been within the medical arena and I have worked as a senior staff nurse, ward sister and as ward manager on an acute medical ward for older people. Care for others has been and always will be my core value, and that includes care for my colleagues as well as patients.

Sue Lillyman MA, BSc (Nursing), RGN, RM, DSPN, PGCE (FAHE)
Faculty Head of Quality Assurance, Faculty of Health and Community Care, University of Central England

Having qualified as a registered general nurse in 1980 and as a midwife in 1983, I worked in various areas, including intensive care, gynaecology and care of the elderly, and rehabilitation and acute medicine until entering nurse education in 1989. Having transferred with the Colleges of Nursing into the University of Central England, I worked as a senior lecturer within the Personal Development Unit for the Faculty of Health and Community Care and in 1997 took up my current role as Faculty Head of Quality Assurance. My teaching responsibilities have been with post-registration nurses undertaking diploma, degree and masters courses in nursing and collaborative community care for healthcare workers. Specialist areas of interest for me include care of the elderly, reflective practice, competence in practice, critical thinking and professional issues. I am soon to complete a PhD at University College, Worcester on the impact of reflection on nursing work.

Dorothy Parsons ONC, SRN, SCM, ENB 998, ACLS,
Dip HE in Organisation of Healthcare, BA Ed (Hons)
Reflective Practice
Sister in an Accident and Emergency Department

I started nursing in 1971, since which time I have worked both in the UK and abroad, from Sutton Coalfield to Saudi Arabia, but always in accident and emergency. I have served my time in management and as a clinical nurse specialist. I have got the T-shirt. I am now where I want to be — in the UK, in the Alexandra Hospital in Redditch, and back with hands-on nursing. Accident and emergency is the front line in patient care. Experience, training and personal development has made me the professional I feel I want to be.

Gail Parsons RGN
Orthopaedic Liaison Sister

I qualified in 1982 as a registered general nurse, orthopaedics being my chosen speciality. I spent ten years as a ward manager on a busy selective orthopaedic unit, and during this time I was seconded to undertake Trust Project Work as part of my personal development objectives. Trust projects included implementing new procedures for working within the x-ray department, workload analysis, and implementing a Trust policy for handling violence and aggression in the workplace. I am now orthopaedic liaison sister in an assessment unit where I undertake holistic patient assessment, health promotion and education. I have recently commenced an MSc in Health Sciences at Birmingham University with a vision of becoming a specialist practitioner.

Dawn Pattison RGN, City and Guilds 730 Teaching Cert,
ISM Dip in Management, BA Ed (Hons) Reflective Practice
Ward Manager — Elderly care medicine ward

I qualified as an RGN in 1989 and worked on a female general surgical ward for two years before moving into general medicine. I successfully achieved the post of ward sister on a medicine ward, prior to assisting in the establishment of an emergency assessment unit for medical patients. I am currently working as ward manager on an elderly care medicine ward. I am interested in the continuing improvement of the knowledge and skills of my colleagues and myself, and hence I value the use of reflective practice along with clinical supervision as a means of fulfilling this goal and also to improve patient care.

Helen Roden RGN, B Sc (Hons), Dip Man, Dip Nurs
HMR, Training and Development Services

I qualified as a registered nurse in 1986 and spent the first two years of my career within intensive and coronary care. I then worked within medicine, firstly gaining experience in the role of primary nurse on a general medical ward. My career progressed within medical specialities. Eventually I gained the post of ward manager. After this, I decided to pursue my interest in developing nursing and gained a post as practice development nurse. I have a strong belief in personal development and my main areas of interest are clinical supervision, lifelong learning and clinical leadership.

Clare Weatherhead RGN, BA Ed (Hons) Reflective Practice
Deputy Sister, Accident and Emergency

I qualified as a registered general nurse in 1991 and commenced my professional career on an acute medical ward before changing speciality to work in accident and emergency. At present I am a deputy sister working in a district general accident and emergency department. Practice within the department is to provide quality care on a 24-hour basis to any patients presenting themselves to the department with conditions ranging from minor to serious physical and psychosocial complaints. My role is to provide a high quality of nursing care whilst also providing effective management of staff and resources. Having worked in the accident and emergency speciality for six years, I have developed a particular interest in resuscitation, including the management of major trauma. I am a member of the Trust's Resuscitation Committee and have recently completed a BA Ed (Hons) degree in Reflective Practice at University College, Worcester.

Acknowledgements

We would like to thank Sue Hampton and Hazel Alley of the Policy into Practice Research Centre at University College, Worcester for their patience, skilfulness and professionalism in helping us to prepare this manuscript. We also owe a debt of thanks to the many colleagues who have listened to our ideas about a book of this kind, have generously given of their time, made us 'think again' about clinical supervision and shared their wisdom about it with us. Particular thanks are extended to colleagues associated with the West Midlands Clinical Supervision Development Network and particularly Neil Brocklehurst, June Patel, Sandra Hulme, Karen Deeny, Carol Dinshaw, Ruth Hawksford and Ruth Hardie for their vision, energy and commitment to making clinical supervision a meaningful, lived reality for healthcare colleagues. Those who have contributed to this book are special people. Thank you for accepting our invitation to write and for being prepared to share your work with a wider audience. We hope you feel proud of what you have achieved.

Tony Ghaye and Sue Lillyman
September, 1999

Introduction. Colleague-centred care: The re-framing of clinical supervision

Tony Ghaye

In the White Papers, *The New NHS: Modern, Dependable* (DoH, 1977) and *A First Class Service: Quality in the New NHS* (DoH, 1998), there is a clear emphasis on improving the quality of care, treatment and healthcare services through an application of the principles and processes of clinical governance. This is to be the new 'work order'. The papers are full of what promises to be a new wave of clinical, managerial and educational buzz-words. Within this developing context lies clinical supervision. It is important that we ask ourselves how we think it fits within clinical governance; how the two can work together in some way to ensure safe and accountable practice. This book attempts to do just this by trying to examine different conceptions of clinical supervision, the ways that individuals and groups have attempted to explore these in practice, and how these two things are motivated by a desire to improve the quality of healthcare provision.

Talk about clinical supervision often suffers from too much meaning. This occurs when we simply assume that the meaning and significance of it is unproblematic. A common illustration of this is where clinical supervision is advanced as some kind of recipe for solving a wide range of 'problems' and thus serving many functions. These functions might be 'clinical', 'managerial', 'educational', 'supportive', and so on. Clinical supervision can also be seen as having too little meaning. Here shared meanings and values are typically more apparent than real. This is not a good basis from which to try to implement clinical supervision. Then there is a third problem: if we do not recognise and address the ambiguity of the term and the surveillance tactics that it connotes; if we do not try to 'customise' and own it in some way, then we may fall for the agendas of others that we might otherwise have rejected on the grounds that they are in fact manipulative, managerialist and oppressive. The chapters in this book illustrate, in various ways, the important difference between being controlled by and being in control of clinical supervision.

The late 1990s is a critical period in the evolution of clinical supervision. Although promising in many ways, its widespread application is problematic. Clinical supervision is being shaped and reshaped. It is difficult at times to discern its different underlying values base; values that might lead to real enhancement of identity and action and to a restructuring of workplaces, or values that fundamentally leave the cultures and arenas of healthcare work largely unchanged. In this sense, the implementation of effective clinical supervision hinges on a paradox. If it is used in the service of more and more healthcare change agendas, it may be in danger of becoming anything and everything. As we know, anything and everything often, in the end, lead to nothing of consequence. I believe it would be unfortunate if the regenerative promise that clinical supervision brings contributed either, on the one hand, to its trivialisation or, on the other, to its subtle co-optation by managers.

A wide variety of case studies and perspectives on clinical supervision are presented in this book. They have enabled two 'golden threads' to weave their way implicitly between the reflective chapters. One is an epistemological thread, the other a methodological one. The former focuses upon what kind of knowledge, if any, is generated through clinical supervision. The latter is about the processes through or by which clinical supervision occurs. For those charged with the responsibility of initiating and sustaining clinical supervision, the message is clear: now is the time to wrestle with the most salient and troublesome questions that our recent experience of it has helped us to frame. Some of these are:

1 What do we want it to mean?
2 What are or should the purposes and consequences of it be?
3 Who is it for?
4 How do we engage with it so that it is an educative experience?
5 How does clinical supervision serve individuals as well as groups?
6 Who benefits from it and who stands to lose?
7 How do the various forms of it contribute to knowledge for and about healthcare?
8 In what ways do its different forms challenge or sustain the status quo?

I would argue that the knowledge question — number 7 — underlies all of the others. It is fundamental to all discussions about clinical effectiveness. The future of clinical supervision will depend upon how this knowledge question is both posed and answered, and this book attempts to address it seriously.

Posing and answering questions about clinical supervision involves a process of constructing and reconstructing meanings and clinical actions. Schon (1983) called this a framing and reframing process. New knowledge and improved action is only possible by learning through the reflective conversations we have with each other as we explore each other's confusions, anxieties, appreciations and achievements. Perhaps after reading this book you might feel that some new thinking and practice is needed if clinical supervision is to be a relevant, lived experience for healthcare professionals. 'Holistic patient-centred care is often regarded as the quintessence of nursing practice' (Ellis, 1999, p.296). I believe that we should actively consider the notion of 'holistic colleague-centred care' as being the quintessence of clinical supervision. This re-framing of the meaning of clinical supervision invites us to reconsider the kind of healthcare professionals that we are; how we try to live our values out in our practice and what we learn from this. It is fundamentally about how we care for others and how they care for us. This conception is fuelled and energised by reflective practices. It is a conception that, in an era of accelerating change, might give us the chance to engage in meaningful work. It might just serve to develop more collaborative working environments of mutual commitment and trust. Of course, I may well be living in cloud-cuckoo-land here! It is not a prediction or even a reality, but it is a hope. A 'holistic colleague-centred care' view of clinical supervision may not lead to clinical areas being more deeply meaningful and fulfilling than the old ones, but such a view may help individuals and groups to be more 'in control' of their own destinies; more able to think for themselves and to question the means and the ends of healthcare work. Our professionalism and freedom depend on this. Such a view may even serve to empower us (Ghaye, 2000). Indeed, what sort of freedom and empowerment do we have if we cannot question the vision, values and goals of the new work order set out in the government White Papers cited at the start of this *Introduction*?

References

Department of Health (1997) *The New NHS: Modern, Dependable.* HMSO, London

Department of Health (1998) *A First Class Service: Quality in the New NHS.* HMSO, London

Ellis S (1999) The Patient-centred care model: holistic/multiprofessional/reflective. *Br J Nurs* **8**(5): 296–301

Ghaye T (2000) Empowerment through reflection: Is this a case of the Emperor's new clothes? In: Ghaye T, Gillespie D, Lillyman S eds (2000) *Empowerment Through Reflection: The narratives of healthcare professionals.* Quay Books, Mark Allen Publishing, Salisbury

Schon D (1983) *The Reflective Practitioner: How professionals think in action.* Basic Books, New York

1

Sowing the seeds of clinical supervision

Helen Roden

In the Bible, in Matthew chapter 13, we are told the parable of the sower:

> *A farmer went out to sow his seed. As he was scattering the seed, some fell along the path, and some the birds came and ate it and some fell on rocky places.... . Still other seeds fell on good soil, where it produced a crop.*
>
> (New International Version, 1979, p.19)

'I don't need to talk to anyone about it, I'm fine,' I snapped back at Sister after she had very calmly enquired if I was all right. This exchange took place about a couple of days after a very difficult case conference to discuss the possible discharge of a young patient for whom I had cared, in the role of primary nurse, over a period of four months. The case conference had been difficult — the patient's consultant, her physiotherapist and occupational therapist did not feel it was appropriate for her to be discharged, but I was acting the role of the patient's advocate and therefore repeatedly stated her case: 'She wants to be discharged'. When I had finally accepted that they were not listening, I invited my patient and her partner to join the meeting and supported them in stating their wishes. I challenged the consultant and I disagreed with the therapists. The meeting left me traumatised, with strong feelings of being undervalued, angry, upset, and questioning the value of the role of primary nurse and the worth of advocacy.

It was, perhaps, the anger that eventually drove me to 'unload' those feelings. An hour spent deconstructing the case conference meeting later, examining my professional values and receiving constructive and positive feedback left me feeling more positive about my role. I was now able to see the outcomes of the meeting more clearly and had a wealth of ideas about what the next steps could be in reaching a satisfactory conclusion to ensure the patient had an early discharge. My belief in clinical supervision was born.

The value of what subsequently became regular, one-to-one clinical supervision sessions is hard to quantify on a sheet of paper. The opportunity to reflect on my practice and to grow; the warm feeling of knowing that someone cared enough to give me time; the hope that these sessions provided for us nurses as professionals; the maturity it took to admit that I had not always got it quite right; the thought of knowing that someone would 'climb in there with me' when the going got tough — all these factors reflect just a glimpse of the value clinical supervision held for me as I worked within the role of primary nurse and, eventually, ward sister.

Although I no longer work within the clinical environment, my belief in the value of clinical supervision is stronger than ever before. This belief has enabled me to accept readily the challenge of exploring the feasibility of implementing clinical supervision for nurses across the whole organisation — a district general hospital. On reflection, if I had fully understood the complexity and enormity of the task that lay ahead of me, I may not have accepted the challenge so readily. However, a vision with belief is a powerful combination in ensuring success.

This chapter tells the story of the real-life issues for one organisation attempting to tackle the implementation of clinical supervision. It endeavours to make the reader aware of the successes of implementation, but also shares the dilemmas and problems that have been part, and in some instances continue to be part, of the story. The story is told from my own perspective and therefore may not always reflect the views of others within the organisation or, indeed, of the organisation itself. Finally, the chapter concludes with a reflective account of my own personal journey through the implementation of clinical supervision.

A vision is born — where were we then?

The starting point, back in 1994, for clinical supervision within the organisation, was the desire of senior nurse managers to find out more about clinical supervision: What was this thing called clinical supervision? What could it offer to nurses? How eaxctly did one 'do' clinical supervision? Having agreed to take the lead role for clinical supervision, I immediately began to reflect on my own experiences. These had a very practical focus, with time spent as a supervisee, supervisor and facilitator but with little underpinning knowledge.

The starting point, therefore, was a literature review that revealed a broad array of models, definitions, frameworks and conflicting evidence about staff and patient benefits. The enormous amount of literature thus reviewed created more questions than it did answers in response to the original questions posed. I knew that all this information had to be processed and chose reflection as the vehicle to achieve this. I reflected on the many conversations that I had had in the different roles I had carried out within clinical supervision. These reflections served as a sieve enabling the gathered information to be filtered; retaining the material that 'made sense' and which related to the organisation, and allowing the rest to drain away into a vat for safe storage to be used at a later date if needed.

The organisation's vision of clinical supervision in 1994 was not the vision that exists in present-day 1999. The vision has moved on. In the beginning it was something that belonged only to a few and could be held in one hand; now it belongs to many. A vision is hard to describe, and words may fail to capture what happens in the organisation but is not always easily visible. In an attempt to give the reader a flavour of the vision, I draw the following analogy. A poppy seed, if planted and nurtured — given the right elements: warmth, light, time, encouragement and patience — grows. The seed develops slowly at first, growing first one set of leaves and then another and another, ceaselessly pushing upwards to reach towards the sun. With continued nurturing the flower head appears, remaining tightly closed at first but eventually opening to reveal a huge, bright, vibrant flower which reflects the light, sways gently in the breeze and attracts nothing but praise. As the flower matures, it sows its own seeds. Some fall in close proximity to itself, but many are carried further away. In a relatively short space of time, where once had stood a single poppy, there now stands a whole meadow full.

The vision was born — the poppy seed was planted. I held the belief that a small number of nurses could develop their skills, so enabling them to become clinical supervisors and provide support and guidance for a further small group of nurses. Initially, the vision was shared by only a few, but nevertheless it was a sufficiently powerful vision to support a pilot project. The pilot was incredibly successful. It consisted of intensive preparation for six nurses over a period of two months and culminated in the provision of clinical supervision for twelve nurses. *Table 1.1* on *page 4* provides an outline of the preparation programme. The evaluation of the pilot project, which included data gathered from both supervisors and supervisees, was totally positive. The seeds had grown and each had a flower head waiting to burst open. I now had a belief that it might be possible to prepare a sufficient number of nurses to take on the role of supervisor and to provide clinical supervision for all the nurses working within the department and wards involved in the pilot — was this possible? It seemed too good to be true!

Table 1.1	Outline of the preparation programme for six nurses involved in the pilot project
Questions discussed:	• What is clinical supervision? • What are the benefits and purpose of clinical supervision? • What are the qualities needed by supervisors? • What is the role of the supervisor?
Items developed:	• a definition • a framework • documentation sheet • a contract.
Issues explored:	• the role of values • relationships • reflective conversations • critical incident analysis.

And so the vision grows — the dilemmas and problems

There is an inherent risk in becoming too wrapped up in the success of the project; of recounting the story as a totally positive account. Reality, however, is a story with dilemmas and problems. The specific dilemmas and problems associated with the implementation of clinical supervision within this organisation are probably no different from those experienced by others attempting to surmount this huge task. Some of the problems are history, some are happening now, whilst others remain as a persistent irritation that disappears, only to reappear somewhere else rather like a mole that decides to make its home under your lawn: whilst celebrating the victory of banishing the mole from your back lawn you stumble over the mound of earth it has created on the front lawn! Other dilemmas remain unresolved like a red wine stain on the carpet which, despite numerous attempts at removal, remains.

The dilemmas and problems are listed opposite:

- 'Ownership or support? You cannot expect both!'
- 'It's great training, but can you do it in less time?'
- 'So you've attended the training, why aren't you providing any clinical supervision?'
- 'Something is better than nothing!'
- 'Will you be my clinical supervisor?'
- 'What else can we do to get them on board?'

Each of these dilemmas and problems will now be discussed in turn, with the reader being made aware of those that were resolved and those that remain. The dilemmas and problems tell the story and explain how the vision grew from a few seeds into a meadow more than half full of poppies.

'Ownership or support? You cannot expect both!' — Not everyone has the same vision

The answer to the question: 'Would you swap senior management support for ownership of clinical supervision by nurses?', perhaps appears to reduce this issue to something far from constituting a major dilemma. The knowledge, however, that many of the executive and senior management team remain oblivious to the concept of clinical supervision, its benefits for staff (Wilkin, 1988; McEvoy, 1993; Faugier, 1995), its potential benefits for patients (Kayberry, 1992; Bishop, 1994; Hallberg, 1994), and its ability to increase job satisfaction and reduce sickness (Butterworth and Faugier, 1992; Skoberne, 1996; Palson *et al*, 1994) still provides a challenge at times. The answer to the opening question is that ownership of clinical supervision by practitioners within the organisation appears to be a far more important factor than is total support from managers. However, it would be naive to believe that managerial support is something which could be ignored; undoubtedly there is a need for both.

From a management perspective there may arise an issue of credibility within clinical supervision. Butterworth *et al*'s (1997) recent study is one of a few that fail to provide substantive tangible evidence to support the view that clinical supervision reduces sickness and has a positive effect on patient outcomes. The absence of such evidence unfortunately reduces the possibility of mounting a convincing argument to support supervision. In a culture which actively encourages evidence-based medicine and research-based decision-making, the clear necessity for evidence is becoming increasingly important.

This issue would perhaps provide a greater challenge for the organisation if practitioners were requesting large sums of money for the implementation of clinical supervision. Without tangible evidence, it is quite impossible to measure the outcomes or to demonstrate cost-effectiveness and value for money, again reducing the bargaining power of practitioners to fight for the need to have supervision in place. The organisation has, in effect, implemented clinical supervision without the need to invest large sums of money, perhaps in turn precipitating a view that clinical supervision is of minimal importance.

In reality there appears to be what amounts to a 'keeping quiet'. If nurses shout too loudly about clinical supervision, thus attracting lots of attention, someone may actually ask: 'When are the nurses finding time for this?' 'How much is this costing us?' The present challenges and pressures facing nurses within the organisation appear to be forcing senior nurses to discuss clinical supervision in depth with their senior managers, and its inclusion within the directorate business plan might reflect this. However, I feel this development is like a double-edged sword. Undoubtedly it is a positive move in terms of accepting that nurses deserve and need clinical supervision, but in direct contrast to this is the knowledge that practitioners will have no other choice but to enter into more discussions with management colleagues about cost, benefit and time associated with clinical supervision.

This dilemma will then, perhaps, become one that 'sits' with senior nurses and their ability to convince senior managers of the value of supervision without having any measurable outcomes to support their arguments. There are, of course, some risks involved in giving total support to supervision without having supporting evidence for it. I would suggest, however, that the risks involved in ignoring supervision are greater. Carthy (1994) states that evidence of the failure to provide supervision is already apparent in wards and departments, manifesting itself in disillusionment, low morale, mediocre performance, poor motivation and fractious relationships between colleagues and managers.

'It's great training, but can you do it in less time?' — As the vision evolved, so did the training

After the preparation programme for practitioners involved in the pilot, a series of clinical supervision days were set up for other nurses who were interested. This, for many practitioners, was their first introduction to clinical supervision, others had some knowledge from having read recent literature, and a few had some experience from being a supervisee in a clinical supervision relationship. These initial training days covered the following issues:

- What is supervision?
- What are the benefits?
- the role of the supervisor
- relationships
- values.

By and large, these training days were evaluated positively. The participants felt informed and positive about supervision, but many questioned how realistic it was. One theme reappearing throughout the evaluation comments was the belief that the information given in the day could be condensed into a half-day session: 'It's great training, but can you do it in less time?' I found this request unbelievable.

On reflection I discovered that I had naively held a belief that this day would, of itself, stimulate nurses to undertake the role of clinical supervisor. Although this was true for a small minority of them — predominantly those more experienced nurses who had been supervisees themselves, for the majority this was not the case. This fact helped to make sense of the request for the training to be condensed into half a day. The handful of nurses who did eventually undertake the role of clinical supervisor benefited from the afternoon session which touched on values and roles, but the majority who didn't want this session appeared to represent the nurses who didn't, at that time at least, see themselves undertaking, or even feel themselves equipped to undertake, the role of clinical supervisor. These factors provided some solid reflective material that enabled the whole issue of training to be reviewed.

It was very clear that the initial day had served successfully as an awareness-raising day for the majority who attended, but that it had not fully equipped those who wished to carry out the role of clinical supervisor with the necessary skills. Review of the training resulted in two firm actions: the first being to condense the clinical supervision day to a half-day awareness-raising session, and the second being to review totally how training would be provided for the nurses wanting to carry out the role of clinical supervisor.

The organisation had an opportunity to participate in a county-wide 'Train the Trainer' programme to prepare nurses to take on the role of clinical supervisor. Some of the participants formed a 'clinical supervision implementation team' which, as its first task, set about redesigning the training. Cutcliffe and Proctor (1998) suggest that if:

> ... *nurses receive insufficient or inappropriate training in supervision, the quality of the supervision that they then provide is unlikely to be capable of producing measured change, indicating improvement in supervisees' mental well-being or improvements in the care they provide.*

A three-day programme was planned which aimed to cover, in depth, all the issues which would ensure that nurses were well prepared to undertake the role of clinical supervisor. *Table 1.2* provides an outline of the programme.

Table 1.2:	Outline of the preparation programme for six nurses involved in the pilot project
Day 1	• What is clinical supervision, its purpose and benefits? • models of supervision and the organisational philosophy • professional values and their relationship to supervision.
Day 2	• reflective practice, including reflective conversations • small group work, to have a go at a supervisory role • legal aspects of clinical supervision • administrative issues, including documentation and reflective diaries.
Day 3	• dealing with difficult situations, including role-play by faculty members to demonstrate good practice • small group work, to have a go at a supervisory role • exploratory session to discuss how it feels to be a supervisor • getting started with supervision: the way forward.

A number of three-day courses have been provided. To date these have been very successful, with positive evaluations but, inevitably, the question came: 'It's great training, but can you do it in less time?' The question came from two sources: firstly from part of the course faculty team who wanted to continue to be part of clinical supervision training but who had huge operational management responsibilities; secondly from the senior nurses and ward managers throughout the organisation who supported clinical supervision but who could not release staff for a three-day course. It feels like a chicken-and-egg situation. Nurses are under a lot of pressure which increases the need for supervision but also dramatically reduces their availability for training. Is there a compromise?

'Compromise' is the right word. The knowledge that the role of clinical supervisor is no easy task, and that quality supervision is dependent upon the skills and abilities of the supervisor (Faugier, 1995; Cutcliffe and Proctor, 1998; Hawkins and Shohet, 1991), all mixed in with a strong belief that nurses must have clinical supervision available to them, has forced a change. To dig one's heels in and say: 'No, the training cannot be done in less time', would surely result in minimal attendance at the courses, thus reducing the availability of supervisors.

So the present compromise is a two-day course, with a few resulting alterations to the programme and some shortened sessions. Participants who had previously undertaken the course had felt exhausted at the end of each day, and this is likely to be augmented with the redesign. The evaluation process will show how participants respond to the resulting increase in pace, and whether they feel less well-prepared to take on the role once training has finished. The dilemma will remain, however, until some of the operational issues are resolved and so this remains very much as a compromise; something the organisation is living with: 'No, the training cannot really be done in less time but it will be done in less time — at least for now.' The issue of training feels like the mole hole analogy — it goes away, but experience reminds you that it will be back.

'So you've attended the training, why aren't you providing any clinical supervision?' — The vision is not happening fast enough

This problem feels like a red wine stain on the carpet; something you cannot ever completely remove. Some nurses within the organisation have now received clinical supervision training, equipping them to take on the role of clinical supervisor and thus to provide regular supervision for a small number of nurses. Nurses report leaving the training course feeling motivated, enthused and ready to embrace the role. They leave equipped with practical tips about how to get started and where to come for reassurance and support if things are not going well. Whilst no participant to date has ever left a programme saying that they are not the right person to carry out the role, or that they do not feel ready or equipped, this in fact, may represent one of the reasons why some do not proceed to undertake the role of clinical supervisor. Whilst I acknowledge that this group is in the minority, it still represents a dilemma and also reduces the availability of supervisors following each course.

Discussion with participants whom this dilemma affects — the steering group and colleagues throughout the region — reveals a variety of possible explanations. The first of these was in connection with the selection process for the three-day course which was currently one of self-selection. Should there be selection criteria to come on the course? Should participants be interviewed prior to attending the course? Were the 'right' people attending training? The steering group did not feel in a position, or have any desire, to make decisions about who was 'suitable' or not. The answer to the first two questions was a firm 'No'. It was felt that if nurses self-selected themselves for this training they had sound reasons for doing so and attended training with a belief that they would carry out the role. This view was in line with the belief that nurses should take responsibility for their own learning needs and professional development.

The second possible explanation was linked with the issue of support: 'Were the new supervisors receiving enough support?' 'Was a lack of support the reason why they were not carrying out clinical supervision?' The course participants were encouraged to seek a supervisor for themselves if they did not already have one and to contact one of the faculty members if they wished to, at any time. Few course participants sought help in this way and some did not actually seek a clinical supervisor for themselves. The faculty, whilst having many pressures within their own roles, agreed to contact and follow up a number of participants in order to give encouragement and support. This system has proved difficult to keep going at times and, as the number of participants going through training increases, will undoubtedly become impossible to maintain.

The third explanation, explored in the effort to try to understand this problem, was that of clinical pressures. The continual staffing shortages, the increase in patient turnover, and so on, continued to reduce the availability of time. Some of the new supervisors reported time as a factor which prevented them from getting started.

The fourth issue to be considered as an explanation was specifically for new supervisors returning to a clinical area where clinical supervision was less well established. It would appear that those new supervisors who return to areas where clinical supervision is well established have an easier passage in establishing supervisory relationships, with time to carry out supervision and receiving support from other supervisors.

The reality seems to be that the incidence of nurses who have had training but do not then go on to undertake the role, will be a constant one because of the range of aforementioned explanations. It would appear impossible to put the necessary systems in place to prevent, or even reduce, these four factors from occurring. This reality represents a slight annoyance rather than a major dilemma, causing slowing down of the implementation of clinical supervision by reducing the availability of supervisors, rather than halting implementation altogether.

'Something is better than nothing!' — Are the poppies receiving all the nurturing they need?

This issue is, as the previous one, a red wine stain on the carpet that will probably never go away. The ideal world would be the vision fulfilled: all nurses would be able to have regular clinical supervision as often as they needed it, within work time. The faculty team, delivering a completely positive message during training about the importance of supervision, the need to carry it out within work time, the importance of the right environment and the necessity to try not to cancel sessions, have been left feeling almost hypocritical at times, knowing the reality. Reality often represents a somewhat different picture to that of the fulfilled vision. For clinical priorities must always come first; planned supervision sessions are therefore cancelled or happen outside work time or occur in a less than suitable environment and for less than adequate time.

With the vision squarely planted in my mind of supervision for every nurse within the organisation, it has proved difficult to sit back and know that this is happening. There has been a temptation to protest loudly at every opportunity and at every level within the organisation that this is not acceptable and that nurses deserve and need clinical supervision. Protesting loudly has not always attracted positive responses, with senior nurses challenging the level of awareness that educators have of the great pressures within the clinical environment. Not to protest, however, would demonstrate a lack of commitment to clinical supervision and the benefits it brings.

So the protesting will continue until such time as this dilemma is resolved and nurses are not having to compromise their colleagues with what is the very limited time they have available for clinical supervision at present. I personally would never tell nurses to stop giving — or trying to give — clinical supervision, even when it seems impossible to fit in. Something *is* better than nothing.

'Will you be my clinical supervisor?'

The course aims to be interactive, with each of the participants having an opportunity to question the faculty members about their own experiences of clinical supervision, to observe them in action during role-play and to receive practical advice as well as support and enthusiasm. This has the effect of increasing the popularity and familiarity of the faculty members as 'experts' within clinical supervision. Many participants, perhaps in an immediate desire to find an experienced supervisor, subsequently approach individual faculty members and ask them to be their clinical supervisor. Whilst this is flattering for the faculty, it also causes a dilemma between wanting to support participants and knowing that, realistically, it is unwise to supervise too many people at one time. Each of the faculty members already has some well-established clinical supervision relationships with a number of nurses within the organisation, so they generally encourage the new supervisors to find a different supervisor to give support; suggesting, if necessary, the names of those nurses who have themselves already undertaken the training.

This dilemma stretches right across both individual and group supervision. The organisation has recently identified a separate need to provide group clinical supervision for some areas. As the organisation has, in the past, predominantly used a model of one-to-one clinical supervision, the issue of group supervision is not discussed within training. The faculty members, therefore, are the only people with any experience of group supervision and again find themselves swamped with requests. I recently started some sessions for a group of E grade staff nurses but then, because of work pressures, was unable to continue with the commitment. This was a difficult decision but one based on believing that it was better not to provide the supervision if I was unable to give a total commitment.

This dilemma will, of course, reduce as the number of clinical supervisors increases, and also with the introduction of further training opportunities for group supervision.

'What else can we do to get them on board?' — There are no poppies in part of the field!

Some parts of the organisation have yet to take their first step towards implementing clinical supervision. Clinical supervision within the organisation is completely voluntary, so nurses have total choice about whether or not they want to be a part of it.

This issue is one which can, at times, almost be forgotten as one is swept along with the excitement of the developments and progress in other areas. The reminder of the raw facts usually comes in the form of a distressed nurse who feels that there is no one to talk to about, for example, his or her involvelemt in a recent critical incident. Then, I always feel a temptation to go straight to the ward manager of the area the nurse is working in and ask when he or she is going to 'wake up, smell the coffee' and do something about clinical supervision. By the time I have either provided some 'first aid' for the nurse myself or found another supervisor to provide this service, the desire to take such aggressive action has passed.

Members of the steering group have discussed this issue on several occasions, always asking: 'Is there anything more we can do to get these areas on board with supervision?' In a search for understanding, we reflected on this issue: 'What was happening?' 'Why was this?' 'How were the staff feeling?' 'Why were they feeling like this?' 'What could be done to change this?' Some possible explanations were generated from this reflective exercise:

- suspicion towards clinical supervision — specifically about what it is, who would be doing it and what the benefits are
- scepticism about whether it could really make a difference
- lack of support from ward managers who play a crucial role in the successful implementation of supervision
- the ever-present issue of lack of time.

A great deal of time and effort has been spent in attempting to address these issues. The effort has been in the form of a continual 'chipping away' — when you felt you couldn't go back and say it again because you had explained it three times already, was precisely the time that you did go back and explain again. Just when you declared you had thrown the towel in, a nurse would come to you distressed and asking why they didn't do clinical supervision in her area, and this would be the catalyst that would make you take up the reins once more.

The effort is starting to bring rewards. The last training course for supervisors included a number of participants from one of the areas which to date had done very little to implement clinical supervision.

The moral of this tale must be: 'Don't give up!' There is always something more that you can do in an effort to ensure that nurses have sufficient information to enable them to understand what clinical supervision is and what it can offer them, to have an opportunity to receive training that will enable them to undertake the role of clinical supervisor if desired, and to have the opportunity to be part of a clinical supervision relationship.

Viable clinical supervision — so how does the poppy field look now?

In order to bring the reader up to date with the current situation regarding the implementation of clinical supervision within the organisation, I will return to the vision and the analogy used throughout this account. Ultimately, when the vision is reached, there will be a field full of poppies representing an abundance of clinical supervisors providing supervision for all nurses.

Despite the dilemmas and problems experienced along the way, and those that continue to provide daily challenges, the vision is in sight. The implementation group continues to meet regularly to develop the training programme and to discuss issues that arise. Progress is rapid at present and more training is planned in response to the demand from nurses and their managers. Advanced clinical supervision training, including facilitation of groups, will be offered soon for the more experienced supervisors.

It is true to say that some areas of the field are totally bare, and that the soil has not yet been assessed to establish which nutrients need to be added in order to enable seeds to grow in it. Some seed has been planted on stony ground and more work is needed here to increase the richness of the soil if these seeds are to grow. There are some areas within the field where the seeds, though sparsely planted, are growing slowly. These seeds need continual nurturing to enable them to develop into full-size poppies. Some areas within the field carry poppies in full flower, almost ready to spread their own seed, but the most pleasurable site, however, is the abundance of poppies already in full flower, standing tall and bright and swaying gently in the breeze, casting their seed near and far.

The organisation has now developed a clinical supervision

booklet which is given to every nurse. Clinical supervision forms part of the recently developed Nursing and Midwifery Strategy, and for the first time has been included within the directorate business plans. Clinical supervision is here to stay and is, most definitely, on the agenda.

My personal journey through the vision

My personal journey through the vision has been a journey of discovery. When, back in 1994, I was first asked to implement clinical supervision I had a personal vision; no one ever asked me what that vision was but undoubtedly it was the main driving force throughout the implementation. If anyone had asked what the vision was I would have been able to tell them. What I would have said then, however, is very different from what I would say now about clinical supervision.

In the beginning, my vision of clinical supervision was based on the personal beliefs I held, and reflected my own positive experiences. I believed that clinical supervision was right for nurses, and that both implementing and using it was something which I could do to provide support for my clinical colleagues. The opinion that I held then was fairly simplistic. I had a naive view about the training nurses needed in order to take on the role of clinical supervisor and believed everyone would welcome clinical supervision with open arms.

My present perspective is more strategic. My motivation for continuing to introduce and to support clinical supervision is heavily influenced by my role as an educationalist, my organisational values and such notions as professional self-regulation and lifelong learning. My present vision is not only for my own organisation but for every nurse, and is simply that all nurses must have access to a skilled clinical supervisor, that the relationship should be built on trust and confidentiality and have reflection at its core. The view that I hold now is realistic, being founded on a sound knowledge base and much greater experience.

The journey from the initial vision to the present one involved many steps. I developed a concrete and wide-ranging theoretical knowledge through researching existing texts, and developing a comprehensive network of other individuals who were experts in clinical supervision. I was involved with a number of regional groups examining clinical supervision and investigating training, its implementation and evaluation, and took the lead role in developing a countywide 'Train the Trainer' initiative.

I feel strongly that if I am providing training and development for trainee supervisors, then I have to be a credible supervisor myself. Throughout the journey I have participated actively in a number of increasingly challenging clinical supervision relationships with senior colleagues, facilitated group supervision and was supervised myself throughout this process.

I have grown and developed personally during this journey and my belief in clinical supervision has strengthened as I have watched individual practitioners develop and grow themselves. I believe that this is something nurses must continue to do and that the lack of tangible outcomes (seen as very important by non-clinical managers) must be measured against the experiences of professionals such as myself who have seen the difference clinical supervision makes.

But what is sown on good soil is the man who hears the word and understands it.

(Bible, Matt. 13:3, p.19)

References

Bible (1979) New International Version. International Bible Society, New York

Bishop V (1994) Clinical supervision for an accountable profession. *Nurs Times* **90**(39)

Butterworth T *et al* (1997) *It is good to talk. Clinical supervision and mentorship: An evaluation study in England and Scotland.* School of Nursing, Midwifery and Health Visiting, Manchester University

Butterworth T, Faugier J (1992) *Clinical supervision and mentorship in nursing.* Chapman and Hall, London

Carthy JC (1994) Bandwagons roll. *Nurs Standard* **8**(38)

Cutcliffe JR, Proctor B (1998) An alternative training approach to clinical supervision. *Br J Nurs* **7**(5)

Faugier J (1995) Thin on the ground. *Nurs Times* **91**

Hallberg IR (1994) Systematic clinical supervision in a child psychiatric ward, satisfaction with nursing care, tedium, burn out and the nurse's own reports on the effects of it. *Arch Psychiatr Nurs* **8**(1)

Hawkins P, Shohet R (1991) *Supervision in the helping professions.* Open University Press, Milton Keynes

Kayberry S (1992) Supervision — Support for Nurses. *Senior Nurse* **12**(5)

McEvoy P (1993) A chance for feedback. *Nurs Times* **89**(47)

Palson ME, Hallberg IR, Norberg A *et al* (1994) Systematic clinical supervision and its effects for nurses handling demanding care situations. *Cancer Nurs* **17**(5)

Skoberne M (1996) Supervision in nursing. My experience and views. *J Nurs Management* **4**

Wilkin P (1988) Someone to watch over me. *Nurs Times* **84**(33)

2

Challenging values in clinical supervision through reflective conversations

David Eltringham, Penny Gill-Cripps and Margaret Lawless

Introduction

The nursing profession is undergoing a period of great change. Clinical supervision is increasingly being seen as a necessary and integral part of the development of all nurses, to assist them in coping with change effectively, efficiently and competently.

Clinical supervision has the potential to assist nurses to develop and define theoretical knowledge based on their own practical experience. By actually challenging values, beliefs and assumptions, clinical supervision encourages nurses to think about their practice in new and different ways, and this promotes a deeper understanding about nursing care.

Clinical supervision has gained national support from the NHS Management Executive Document, *A Vision for the Future* (DoH, 1993). Target ten of this document identified that nurses require support in developing their practice and that clinical supervision

> ... is central to the process of learning and to the expansion
> of the scope of practice and should be seen as a means of
> encouraging self-assessment, analytical and reflective skills.

Further prominence was given in the form of a letter from the Chief Nursing Officer (DoH, 1994) which clearly identifies her belief in the value of clinical supervision to safeguard standards, develop professional expertise and deliver quality care. The UKCC, in its *Position Statement on Clinical Supervision for Nursing and Health Visiting* (1996), further endorsed the value of clinical supervision in improving practice and increasing understanding of professional issues. Furthermore, the UKCC identified that clinical supervision is not a managerial system.

The authors of this chapter met as a writing team whilst

studying on the BA Ed (Hons) degree programme in Reflective Practice at University College, Worcester. As an element of our engagement with the task of writing we developed a title that reflected our previous interest in clinical supervision. This piece of work is in the form of a 'reflective conversation' (as identified in *Chapter 4*) about clinical supervision between three nurses with the roles of manager, educationalist and clinician. The structure of the chapter mirrors the structures in a trilogy of texts entitled, *Critical Conversations* (Ghaye and Wakefield, 1993; Plummer and Edwards, 1993; Ghaye, 1996). This conversational form allows two people to express a personal point of view and to respond to each other. In this chapter one of us presents our written views on clinical supervision and offers them to another in the group, in the role of critical friend, for comment. Upon receiving these comments, the original writer makes a response to the thoughts expressed by the critical friend. The complete exchanges that result therefore represent a reflective dialogue between professionals.

> *These conversations represent something of the identities of those engaged in them. They convey a sense of self, a sense of relationship with another and a sense of commitment to understand self, others and the context in which prof-essional practice takes place.*
>
> (Ghaye and Wakefield, 1993, p.x)

David Eltringham, senior nurse — medicine (when writing this chapter)

Initial thoughts about clinical supervision

My experience of clinical supervision began relatively late in my career. As a resuscitation training officer, I was offered some support by a colleague and this developed into a formal clinical supervision relationship. Prior to this experience I had a limited understanding of clinical supervision and was sceptical about its use. The concept map, *Figure 2.1* on *page 21*, illustrates my perception of clinical supervision at that time.

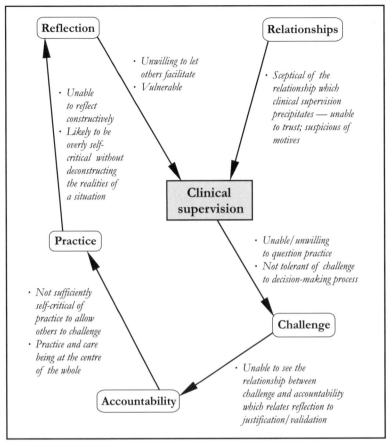

Figure 2.1: Concept map describing David's perspective on clinical
supervision 'then'

My ability to analyse my practice critically has matured, as has my
ability to develop critical and challenging relationships. This is
illustrated for me by the strength of relationship and the level of trust
that I have with my own supervisor. I believe that clinical supervision
is an excellent medium for personal and professional development and
I wholeheartedly advocate its use within my teams. The personal
benefits for me are summarised in the concept map, *Figure 2.2* on
page 22, that illustrates my current feelings about clinical supervision.

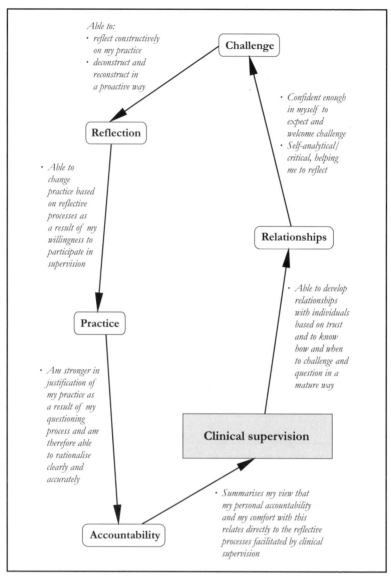

Figure 2.2: Concept map describing David's perspective on clinical supervision 'now'

Target ten from *A Vision for the Future* (DoH, 1993) describes the development of a framework for clinical supervision and also incorporates a definition of clinical supervision (paragraph 3.27). Clinical supervision:

> *... is a term used to describe a formal process of professional support and learning which enables individual practitioners to develop knowledge and competence, assume responsibility for their own practice and enhance consumer protection and the safety of care in complex clinical situations.*

I maintain that there is something of a conflict between the formal definitions that are advocated by such organisations as the NHS management executive on the one hand and the philosophy of clinical supervision in which I believe. The personal motivation for me is the perceived improvement in quality of care for patients, together with the extension of a philosophy of caring into working teams. In other words, the professionals in a clinical supervision relationship, within the organisational boundaries, are themselves being cared for.

For many people the concept of clinical supervision is drawn from the literature of which there is a large volume. *A Vision for the Future* (DoH, 1993) is often a good place to start. I have critically analysed its definition to illustrate the conflict I see arising between the formal definition that many managers may use to initiate the implementation of clinical supervision on the one hand, and a values-based philosophy on the other. I have deconstructed the definition in order to address each part systematically and have then discussed each part in relation to my own professional values.

Formal process

I believe there must be a formal structure in place within an organisation to support clinical supervision. This then ensures that boundaries are appropriately set and that supervisors and supervisees are clear about the nature of those boundaries. In addition, a framework that is approved by the organisation gives credibility to the notion of support for supervision within a busy operational area.

Professional support

I believe that it is appropriate for professionals to seek advice from one another and to challenge practice, so creating a culture of reflection on practice. 'Support' as a term is difficult to define and could be interpreted differently by different individuals.

Learning and development of knowledge

I believe that clinical supervision, through challenging practice, allows an individual to learn and to grow.

Competence

I believe that there is no such thing as absolute competence, but that a practitioner can be more or less competent depending upon their level of skill and experience.

Assuming responsibility for own practice

I believe that nurses are increasingly responsible for delivering clinical care and are becoming more and more autonomous in the application of their practice. An important means of maintaining clinical safety in autonomous practice must be through critical reflection upon practice, and clinical supervision by its nature facilitates this. Accountability in nursing practice has not changed in that registered nurses remain accountable within four arenas of accountability (Dimond, 1995, p.5). Nurses need to be ever-mindful of this, and the ability of individuals to account for and to justify practice is strengthened by challenge and debate.

Safety of care

I believe that through challenging and questioning practice; by raising the profile of accountability; and by debating the application of values of care professionally, patient care remains safe and considered whilst also being innovative, creative and individualised.

By taking the definition apart in this way it is possible to see how the values and beliefs of individual interpretation can be applied to make it come alive. To support the argument for clinical supervision, it is important to identify some of the potential constraints a manager may face in implementing a framework of clinical supervision.

It must be made quite clear that clinical supervision is not a management tool and that the supervisor/supervisee relationship is absolutely confidential. Best and Rose (1996, p.84) refer to the 'right to privacy', and I wholeheartedly support this, with one exception. As registered nurses we have an obligation to protect the public, and I apply the same principles to maintaining confidentiality: an accountable practitioner may breach confidentiality only if it is judged that this would be in the interests of patient safety (UKCC, 1992). A better approach to this difficult problem is the offer of support for an individual by their supervisor when facing such a dilemma. This would mean that in only the most serious situations would a breach of confidence be necessary.

The view that managers can use clinical supervision as a management tactic is one that I cannot support, having said that I understand some of the worries about this. The very phrase 'clinical supervision' implies a bureaucratic approach, and it needs to be sold carefully to potential participants so that it does not become a threat but is seen as a positive and proactive way of dealing with the difficult situations which most practitioners face on a day-to-day basis. Interestingly, my own experience reflects this in a very positive way. Initially I was very sceptical about the process of clinical supervision and was won over with careful explanation together with gentle initial experiences. It is interesting to reflect that the person who fulfilled this role was my manager for a considerable period of time.

Reply to David's first piece of work: Penny's reflections

The most striking aspect of this perspective is the excitement with which you write and the energy that you pour into the process of clinical supervision both for yourself and for others. You describe this well within your 'then' concept map. The words you use to describe your initial feelings 'then' are 'vulnerable', 'sceptical', 'unwilling' and 'unable to trust', which are words that I used myself back then. These words have since disappeared and been replaced by other words of growth, challenge, development, confidence and willingness to accept.

The reception I first received when I initially began to raise awareness of supervision in theatres was very similar to your first reaction, and so this transformation is encouraging for me as an educator because I now feel that it is possible to increase motivation and ask others to consider supervision as a tool to help them in their practice. Throughout your piece you write passionately about the concept of clinical supervision, your role in its implementation and the growth you have found for yourself within a clinical supervision setting. You advocate clinical supervision for all your staff and you have written this into your objectives for the smooth running of your directorate and the support of your staff. You are well prepared for the changes and hard work that lie in front of you. However, I do feel that you have an extremely difficult task on your hands in balancing the needs of your nurses and the needs of the service. I would like to ask you, as a manager, if you give any support to the idea that the UKCC should be more proactive in introducing supervision for nurses (Farrington, 1996, p.716).

The position paper from the UKCC firmly insists that clinical supervision is '... not to be a mandatory requirement for nurses and health visitors...', but may be looked at again 'if the need arises' (UKCC, 1996). It is clear that 'Clinical supervision will play an increasingly important part in ensuring safe and effective practice...' — a factor that you declare is one of your main priorities. Perhaps the idea, then, of a mandatory statement or more emphasis and weight from the UKCC would make the task of implementation for you, as a manager, a great deal easier. As both a practitioner and a manager this may have an uncomfortable feel to it but, with the ever-increasing workload, how are you going to convince nurses who are already stretched that they need to give time and commitment to this process? You are, however, an excellent role model and educator. I believe you are very self-aware and also a charismatic leader. I feel that with these qualities you will earn the respect of many.

The UKCC is also clear that supervision should not be used as a management tool or performance review, which point you reiterate in your script. I would like to ask how you intend to change attitudes and to gain support from the Trust and its managers. I believe that without the support of management both in allowing time for clinical supervision and also in the implementation phase, the possibility of support for all nurses through this medium is limited.

I realise that the needs of the patients and of the service are paramount, whichever way of working is followed, and we seem to be in agreement here but:

> ... *changes in the underlying culture leading to super-vision as a valued part of the work are needed for it to succeed. Simply paying lip-service to the idea without real commitment to and understanding of the task of supervision is unlikely to be of use...*

(Kaberry, 1992, p.39)

One of your tasks is to make nurses '... work smarter rather than harder...', as stated by Nicklin (1995, p.24), who goes on to say, '... clinical supervision should improve competence, confidence and efficiency...' and again, from your own words, this is what you see as your ultimate goal.

You conclude your perspective by suggesting that the initial worries about clinical supervision perhaps stem from the actual words themselves and each individual's interpretation of them. I have often thought about this myself and would rather use the term 'clinical support' instead of 'clinical supervision'.

David's reply to Penny's comments

Thank you, Penny. It is very perceptive of you to draw on my initial views about clinical supervision in the context of this reflective conversation, particularly as you also describe the passion with which I now write. I think that for me there has been an increase in self-awareness through clinical supervision, and the discovery of a piece of myself which allows me to ask the right questions of myself.

There exists a complex debate which you have uncovered. As a manager I have an obligation to care for my team. The team consists of over 120 people and I cannot possibly care directly for them all. The opportunity for members of staff to access clinical supervision is my way of offering care. I simply cannot agree with Farrington's statement (1996, p.716) that clinical supervision should, perhaps, be a mandatory requirement. I believe that its imposition is counter-productive. I do not believe that there is a role for the UKCC in making clinical supervision compulsory. The value of clinical supervision for me is that it belongs to me. I chose my supervisor, I use my reflective diary to set the agenda and I treat the sessions in absolute confidence. I feel no threat in discussing many potentially threatening and sensitive issues. I believe that compulsory sessions would compromise my freedom. One of my concerns as a manager is that we work in an arena where evidence-based practice is becoming a requirement. There is little evidence to support clinical supervision in practice by outcome measurement (Butterworth, 1997). My instinct tells me that there is an intrinsic value in providing support for professionals in this manner and that we should persevere in attempting to collect and present more persuasive qualitative data.

In terms of my persuading my own team to adopt clinical supervision, I have begun to use a number of strategies:

1　I have actively participated in the development of a framework for clinical supervision across the Trust, from within the Trust steering group.
2　I have written the objective into the directorate business plan, thereby gaining the support of the clinical directorate and the directorate manager.
3　I actively participate in clinical supervision as a supervisor and a supervisee and believe that this constitutes role modelling.
4　I have actively established a clinical supervision process in areas of the directorate dealing with crisis, and will continue to do this in areas which will, from time to time, experience crisis.

I think it is interesting that you ask two questions which I now choose to answer as one. You ask how I will influence my team and persuade them to adopt clinical supervision without imposing it, and also how I will influence other managers in the Trust to support the implementation of clinical supervision. The team, for me, includes the other managers within the Trust and I see this as a broad change management exercise. My experience suggests that my colleagues in other areas do not have the same views about clinical supervision as my own, but I believe that managers who are 'non-believers' must put their views to one side and allow their teams to become involved. Perhaps my own experiences will be useful in providing support for them through this process. I would suggest, however, that it is very difficult to present a convincing argument without evidence of its benefits both for individuals and on patient care.

Penny Gill-Cripps — practice development nurse

Initial thoughts about clinical supervision

My own introduction to clinical supervision came in 1996 when, as part of my role as practice development nurse, I attended an in-house three-hour session entitled, 'Introduction to Clinical supervision'. The work I do here within the Trust is concerned with the support of registered practitioners, both within the clinical area and in their own personal development. I knew very little about clinical supervision at that time, but my initial thoughts were that this support should become an integral part of clinical practice. Following this session I began asking for invitations from the clinical areas to talk to nurses in order to increase their awareness of the concept of clinical supervision and to stress the benefits for both practitioners and practice.

My own clinical background is surgical, and so I concentrated my efforts within the surgical area and theatres. I was very surprised by the reception I was given there. The motivation and morale of the nurses were very low at the time because of threats of department closure, the pressures of workload and diminished staff numbers. Consequently there was very little excitement or willingness to participate in what many nurses viewed as another 'bandwagon' to climb aboard. There were also cries of 'here we go again' and 'we are already doing this and it does not help' and of course the ever-present 'when do we get the time?'

Although I had not expected to change the situation overnight, I was disappointed by the lack of interest and the distrust that was shown. I can see now that this resistance was a reaction to change and the fear of what change might bring.

My sessions were a summary of the workshop that I had attended, and lasted only an hour. I concentrated on the senior staff and completed sessions for E, F and G grade nurses who had the experience to deal with most aspects of theatre work.

It is disappointing to look back now over twelve months to find that very few, if any, of those nurses have either become supervisors or found supervision for themselves. This is a situation I have found difficult to come to terms with because theatre is a very intensive and demanding area and I have often been present when staff are clearly upset over personality and practice issues and yet they insist that these pressing problems are not affecting patient care or their own personal growth.

Within the nursing profession there still exists a blame culture and an attitude that asking for support is a weakness and this, I believe, is perhaps why so many nurses in need do not come forward to seek help. I also feel that, in theatre especially, the nurses saw clinical supervision as a threat because of the rumours that '... supervision is a desire to control nurses by manipulating or spying on them' (Castledine, 1994, p.1135).

Perhaps the most difficult aspect concerning the time spent in raising awareness amongst the nurses was their complete mistrust of a concept that could bring them so many benefits if only they were not so reticent about embracing it! After such a disastrous start on the road to implementation, I felt that I needed to reassess my role as educator and facilitator in order to make the implementation of clinical supervision a success. I felt I lacked the knowledge and the skill that I needed to underpin the philosophy of clinical supervision (see *Figure 2.3*). I was extremely grateful, therefore, to be given the opportunity to attend a three-day 'Train the Trainer' course to enable me to fulfil those learning needs.

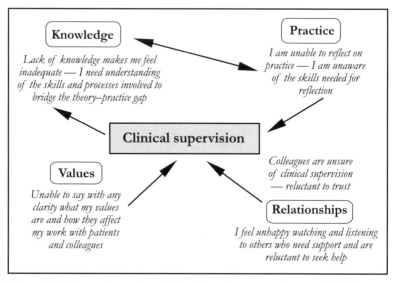

Figure 2.3: Concept map describing Penny's perspective on clinical supervision 'then'

Initially I thought that all that was needed to implement clinical supervision was enthusiasm, and that the laying of emphasis on the benefits for practice and practitioners would 'sell the product'. The knowledge that I have gained during the course has shown me that clinical supervision is much more complex than I first assumed. One of the most thought-provoking aspects of the course has been the realisation that, as a key player in the implementation of supervision and as a prospective supervisor, I need to be very aware of my own skills, capabilities and practice before I can realistically engage my supervisee in productive and supportive interaction. It is important for me to work actively towards becoming a reflective practitioner and to encourage others to do so also. This involves questioning my own practice in such a way that my beliefs, values and attitudes are put under the microscope to be examined (see *Figure 2.4* opposite).

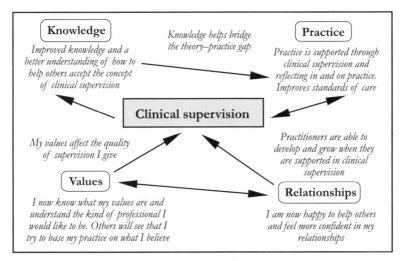

Figure 2.4: Concept map describing Penny's perspective on clinical supervision 'now'

It can be very frightening when, after years of moving gently along, one suddenly has to question one's actions, challenge behaviour, change old habits and adopt different ways of working and thinking.

As a teacher I feel I have the responsibility to help and support nurses through those difficult times; to help them to cope with the feelings of vulnerability that reflection on difficult practice situations may bring. The commitment and hard work that is needed to enable nurses to engage in reflective practice may deter many and push those who 'are already doing it' back to the confines of the coffee shop where they feel safer discussing practice without the difficult and challenging questions. With my new-found knowledge I feel now that I can challenge attitudes and question assumptions and show that by using reflection the rewards far outweigh the discomfort.

Reply to Penny's first piece of work: Margaret's reflections

In your account, you descriptively set the picture of how you envisage clinical supervision acting as a vehicle of support and development — not for yourself, but for the nurses you work with. This immediately makes a statement to me about you, Penny, as a professional. As practice development nurse, I think your concerns are and should be the nurses. The focus for you has moved away from the patient, but you seem to be able to apply the same principles of care to the nurses as you would to a patient. This connects with my own account where I applied the principle of primary nursing and Peplau's model (1988) to my colleagues as well as to my patients. Your unselfish approach of giving to others without considering yourself is typical of many in the nursing profession and it could be the very reason why you have found it so difficult to introduce clinical supervision in theatres. In your account, though you do offer other interpretations, you suggest the explanations firstly of nurses not wishing to be seen as being unable to cope and, secondly, of their perception of clinical supervision as being used as a control mechanism. Your own past experiences within the surgical arena enable you to make a perceptive judgement here which you expertly link to the professional literature.

I was saddened by your recollections of your first attempt to implement clinical supervision. I think you are extremely self-critical. I believe you should not have seen this as failure, but as another step on the learning curve. This links with what you wrote of in a different context in the previous paragraph, that 'within the nursing profession there still exists a blame culture...'. Why did you blame yourself for this first attempt at implementing such a major innovation, and see it as a failure? I would also like to ask you if you yourself are receiving clinical supervision at this stage of your career, to see if you have the opportunity to explore these personal feelings you have towards your practice.

After further reflection you appear to have identified and acted upon your own personal development needs — hence your attendance at the 'Train the Trainer' course to gain the knowledge and skills of clinical supervision. Your reflections portray that you now have a greater understanding of your personal position and influence — the tacit has been made explicit (Ghaye *et al*, 1996, p.7). Your concept maps demonstrate the growth in your maturity from a position of powerlessness to one of liberation and the ability to continue moving forward.

You also believe, as a teacher, that you have a responsibility to 'help and support nurses'. Educationalists must engage in clinical practice to be valued and acknowledged (Ford and Walsh, 1995). I would like to ask you how you see your role within the organisation in achieving this. Will you need to make cultural and policy changes and, if so, how will you manage this? I would also like to ask you about your own personal experiences in the receiving of clinical supervision, in order to explore the congruence between what you say and how you act (Ghaye *et al*, 1996, p.28). You explore both commitment and responsibility. I wonder if, by doing so, you yourself are feeling overwhelmed by the magnitude of this innovation. I know for myself that these are feelings I have experienced myself when considering the numbers of nurses out there — all in need of clinical supervision. However, I believe we should ask ourselves how far our knowledge of supervision and our awareness of the potential impact it could have on practice has contributed to our current feelings.

In your piece there is an outstanding awareness of the need for reflection that connects with my own account and my belief that reflection is the key to effective clinical supervision.

Penny's reply to Margaret's comments

I feel that I should begin by saying 'thank you', Margaret, because having now read your reflections on my work, I am beginning to realise what a reflective conversation looks and feels like (even though it is a written conversation) and, for me, this is an exciting moment. Our conversation does focus on caring values, it does look forward to what will be, interrogates clinical experiences and perhaps most importantly it has enlightened and empowered. I admit that I was feeling disappointed and negative about my initial efforts to introduce clinical supervision but I have now found that I am able to look at those feelings in a different way. Your words are both challenging and supportive, and they have helped me to think in different ways too.

You asked me to consider whether I felt 'overwhelmed by the magnitude of this innovation' (of implementing clinical supervision in the organisation) which was *exactly* how I felt. It was impractical of me to think that just because I said, 'Try clinical supervision, it will make you a more effective practitioner', that nurses would welcome it with open arms. I have looked at change theory in some depth. 'Many nurses are damaged humans as a result of change forced upon them, leaving them able only to react and resent' (Wright, 1989, p.4). I realise that I should have given this statement consideration instead of criticising myself.

You also mention that my focus has moved away from the patient and that I now concentrate my efforts on supporting the nurses. I believe that by helping the nurses within clinical supervision they will become more confident and feel more valued, which in turn will address one of the aims of supervision — to raise safety and quality of care for patients. I have already suggested that clinical supervision will be the process to make this happen and I hope this answers the question: 'Who is caring for us when we are so busy caring for others?'

To answer your question about my own experience of clinical supervision, I must admit here that I was not in a supervision relationship and did not understand the importance of reflection either in practice or on practice at that time. I did not realise that reflection was the key to quality supervision, as indeed you suggest. Through the work I have done on a degree course — the BA Ed (Hons) in Reflective Practice at University College, Worcester — I am now beginning to understand the process of reflection and the power it can exert on practice and practitioners.

To conclude, I would like to answer your question about cultural change. You suggest that I have a part to play within my role in order to bring about this change. I strongly agree with your suggestion but would like to add that I think we *all* play a part in effecting change. The culture within the NHS at the moment is one of 'getting the job done' and I feel that, unfortunately, there is little thought given to those who are 'doing the job'. I feel that attitudes must change too. All too often when practitioners talk about limited resources, staff shortages, pressures of time and workload they are met with replies that are inconsiderate and demoralising. If attitudes do not change then we must take it upon ourselves, as practitioners, to develop our own mechanisms of support and development. I am certain that through a framework of clinical supervision, and as a team, we can begin to put those mechanisms in place.

Margaret Lawless — medical ward sister (when writing this chapter)

Initial thoughts about clinical supervision

As a clinician I was first introduced to the concept of reflective practice when I was a third-year student nurse completing my final placement on a medical ward. As I worked with a senior staff nurse we talked about her recent experience as a student midwife. She told me that, as part of her studying, she was encouraged to keep a reflective diary. We discussed how useful she had found this exercise when she had looked critically at what she was doing. This concept appealed to me as I began to see how reflection-on-practice offered greater awareness and insight into everyday work. My first attempts were very ad hoc and I reflected mainly on incidents that caused me stress and concern. I often went weeks or even months without actually putting pen to paper. The reflections were very much private dialogues with myself, but I know that whenever I did reflect I gained solace and satisfaction.

Clinical supervision was introduced to me four years later when I had become a ward sister on a care of the elderly ward. I had previously worked as a primary nurse endeavouring to deliver individualised, holistic patient care. I had also studied Peplau's model of nursing (1988), with its emphasis on the significance of relationships. As a ward sister, I applied the principles of primary nursing and Peplau's model not only to my patients but also to my ward staff. I recognised that my colleagues were in need of help and support and I saw clinical supervision as a vehicle for providing this.

The NHS Trust in which I work developed a scheme to introduce clinical supervision for its nurses. I was one of the first participants of the ensuing study days which were aimed at raising awareness of clinical supervision and at training clinical supervisors. From this experience I was able to enter into a unique relationship with another ward sister with a similar length of experience to myself — a relationship that could be described as 'peer supervision'. Our relationship was built on respect, trust, openness and a mutual need, and gave us the opportunity both to explore and to reflect on our mistakes, vulnerabilities and values in a safe environment. Our focus was frequently on those issues which caused us stress and anxiety, but we also shared those things that we felt had gone well. We shared experiences that were new to each of us, too. Frequently such experiences then became the experience of the other and, because of our previous explorations and reflections, we felt well prepared. This gave to us a deep sense of satisfaction and comradeship.

My colleague has subsequently moved on elsewhere. However, that experience of peer supervision laid down for me the foundation of a more mature approach which I believe has prepared me to take on the challenge of offering effective supervision for my colleagues, and further enhances my recognition of my own growth and development needs. My support now comes from a person who has guided my decision-making throughout my nursing career. Clinical supervision for me is part of a bigger reflective process. I believe I am now developing a questioning approach; challenging my own values and beliefs, previously so firmly held. I regularly record work incidents in a learning journal, following in it a framework of reflection (Ghaye and Lillyman, 1997) and securing the time to do this possessively — no longer as a chore. I often take these reflections to my clinical supervision sessions. I realise that the majority of the time I have worked things out for myself, but because I have respect for my supervisor, because I value her judgement and because my reflections are not rejected or criticised, I am able to respect and accept my own judgement. In *Figures 2.5* (below) and 2.*6* (opposite) I have attempted to demonstrate this personal growth in 'then' and 'now' concept maps.

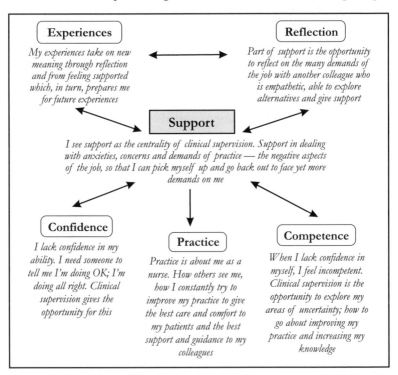

Figure 2.5: Concept map describing Margaret's perspective on clinical supervision 'then'

Clinical supervision for me has been a positive experience; one of growth and of personal development that has increased my self-awareness and has also, I believe, improved my practice. Critically deconstructing incidents that have given me both joy and stress;

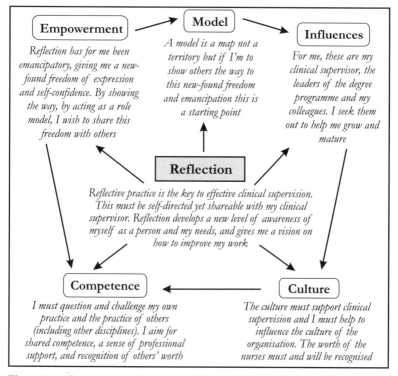

Figure 2.6: Concept map describing Margaret's perspective on clinical supervision 'now'

asking myself why I did it the way I did; exploring alternative methods of working; and then sharing these thoughts with another person whom I respect, has better prepared me to interact with others, whether it be patients or colleagues.

For me, the key to clinical supervision is clearly reflective practice. I believe that, if clinical supervision is to be effective, nurses need to be self-directing and able to sustain their own reflection in order to develop a new level of awareness of themselves as people and of their work. This, I believe, will be a crucial factor when training others to take on the role of clinical supervisor.

Nursing is a demanding as well as a joyful occupation and nurses frequently discuss and reflect on their practice in order to seek guidance and support. Clinical supervision offers a more formal approach that acknowledges the heavy demands of nursing, facilitates reflective practices, and encourages a continuous striving for improvement in the standards of care. Clinical supervision helps me to make sense of what I do and why I do it, and so enables me constantly to push forward my professional boundaries.

Reply to Margaret's first piece of work: David's reflections

Your description of clinical supervision and the experiences you describe which have influenced your present position show a comprehensive and holistic approach to clinical supervision. As a clinician the centrality of care to your practice is evident, not only in the way you describe reflective practices influencing your day-to-day work, but also in the confidence you have in clinical supervision as care for your colleagues. You say, 'I recognised that my colleagues were in need of help and support and saw clinical supervision as a vehicle for providing this.' I would interpret this as an expression of your core motivating values.

I am very interested in your reference to Peplau's work (1988). Nursing is sometimes described as a '... therapeutic relationship' (Forchuk, 1993, p.33). Your reference to Peplau in the context of clinical supervision suggests that, for you, a therapeutic relationship exists within your own experiences of clinical supervision and I absolutely agree with this notion.

Peplau lists and defines four stages in a therapeutic relationship:

- **orientation** during which the individuals in the relationship get to know one another and position themselves
- **identification** where problems are explored and identified
- **exploitation** where the problem itself and its underlying influences are explored, and a plan is developed and implemented to resolve the problem
- **resolution** where the relationship and the growth through the relationship are reviewed, summarised and, ultimately, the relationship is terminated.

I think this reflects the concept of clinical supervision which you own. I wonder if it is possible to superimpose Peplau's theory upon the model which many people use during their clinical supervision experience, namely the normative, formative and restorative model as described by Proctor (1991). It seems reasonable to suggest that each clinical supervision session might see all four of Peplau's stages accessed during the critical encounter, and that the end of the meeting signifies the temporary termination of the relationship.

There may, in addition, be a broader relationship context which also follows Peplau's stages, and this may support the model of supervision used by organisations such as the Probation Service, where supervisors must be changed formally on a regular basis.

Another of your caring values appears to be the belief in reflective practices. You clearly see clinical supervision within the broader context of reflective practice. You see reflection as a central value in your practice and the questioning approach which you say you are developing allows you to feel confident in your own practice. It is interesting that you feel the need to check out your judgement with your supervisor. I can relate to this strongly as this is something I do myself. In describing this phenomenon, I believe you are touching upon the concept of empowerment. Empowerment, I think, is about beliefs and values and having the confidence to put them into practice. Part of this process is being able to articulate those values (Ghaye *et al*, 1996). In complex clinical and management situations it is easy to feel vulnerable when sharing ones values and beliefs with others, particularly if those 'others' are non-nurses. Clinical supervision allows individuals to check out their ideas with a trusted other before being faced with the challenge of sharing them further, and you describe this beautifully.

Your concept maps (*Figures 2.5* and *2.6*) show a change in your position regarding clinical supervision. Initially, support is central to your beliefs and you describe anxieties and concerns in your practice about which you needed reassurance. My own interpretation is that you received the required support and that this is a good example of the success that reflective practice can have in the context of clinical supervision. I say this because your 'now' map places reflection in the centre. The word 'support' does not feature on this map and this suggests to me that perhaps you see reflective practices and clinical supervision as something in which you have confidence. In the broader context, this could apply to the developing professional ethos and the focus of nursing which has changed over recent years. Street (1991) suggests that reflection is a way to:

> *... empower nurses to become fully cognisant of their own knowledge and actions, the personal and professional histories which have shaped them, the symbols and images inherent in the language they use, the myths and the metaphors which sustain them in practice, their nursing experiences and the potentialities and constraints of their work setting.*

I would like to ask you how you feel about this, whether you agree with it and, please, to tell me a little bit more about how you got to where you are now.

Margaret's reply to David's comments

Thank you, David, for your comments.

Yes, I do care. As a clinician, the focus for me is the patient but, as I have gained experience, expertise and awareness, I have been able to take on the bigger picture and to realise that if nurses are to provide quality patient care — which itself is also continually improving — then they need to be healthy individuals themselves, both mentally and physically, and working in a healthy workforce culture. My concern is that this is not always so, and an even greater concern is that nurses do not always realise this. I believe that a questioning approach has got to be cultured if we are to find different ways of doing things and, above all, asserting 'care' as the centrality of nursing — and that includes caring for ourselves and each other. For me, this is what Wright (1997) describes as a 'high-touch' approach which combines both the nurse's caring and therapeutic functions. You are right, David, I do believe that clinical supervision is a 'therapeutic relationship', and that is exactly why I turned to Peplau's (1988) model of care, whose primary focus is on the development of just such a relationship.

This model recognises that life is stressful, but that we also learn and grow from the experiences. When stress overwhelms us we instinctively seek assistance. Peplau's model recognises uniqueness and individuality and that every interaction will be different. I find the model fluid — it allows for creativity by the adoption of certain roles, such as surrogate, resource person, leader, expert, counsellor and teacher. What is required is an acute awareness of self and others, so that the personality can be used to direct the relationship in a way that will maximise the opportunities of the interaction for growth and maturity. This is a huge demand on the nurse, and I believe that few nurses have attained such a level of personal development. It is this that I am striving towards through reflective practice.

I was interested in your thoughts about the four stages to a therapeutic relationship, and in the concept of superimposing Peplau's theory onto the normative, formative, restorative model (Proctor, 1991). I had not made this connection myself, but feel we should explore it further when devising a model of clinical supervision for our own area, in order to devise a flexible framework for diverse healthcare situations.

It was satisfying to me that you use clinical supervision sessions in a similar way to myself — that of checking out judgement with the supervisor. As leading personnel in the introduction of clinical supervision throughout the Trust, I believe we need to demonstrate congruence and stability.

You ask me whether I am touching upon the concept of 'empowerment'. Is this because you, David, have experienced empowerment through being able to communicate your beliefs and values to others? For me it is more a preparation. When a situation occurs which I reflect upon in my learning journal, I feel inclined to share this with my clinical supervisor. The very act of articulation in the clinical supervision session enhances my preparation, allowing me to assert my position in a situation where I previously felt vulnerable. So, yes, perhaps I am touching upon the concept of empowerment.

It was pleasing to me that you interpreted my 'then' and 'now' concept maps in the way you did, because that is exactly what I wished to convey. Writing the concept maps was an extremely useful and exciting exercise, to demonstrate to myself how my beliefs about clinical supervision have developed. I believe we should take serious heed of these concept maps when planning training sessions for future supervisors, in order to recognise where others may be as regards the development of their own clinical supervision experience.

Thinking again

Our consensus is that, if we are to be successful in trying to implement and sustain clinical supervision with our colleagues, we need an agreed philosophy and framework as a starting point when introducing such an enormous innovation. The processes that were involved in preparing this chapter — deconstructing our accounts, writing, and discussing our thoughts and findings with our peers — have provided an opportunity for interaction and enabled further connections to our practice to be made. Perhaps one of the most telling things to be revealed through our reflective conversations and concept-mapping activities is the power of the phrase one of us used one evening, namely: 'the value of clinical supervision for me is that it belongs to me'.

References

Best D, Rose M (1996) *Quality Supervision. Theory and Practice for Clinical Supervisors.* Saunders, London

Butterworth T (1997) *It is good to talk: An evaluation of clinical supervision in England and Scotland.* The University of Manchester, Manchester

Castledine G (1994) What is Clinical Supervision? *Br J Nurs* **13** (21): 1135

Cox (1993) from 'Train the Trainer' course notes

Daley B (1996) Concept maps: Linking nursing theory to clinical nursing practice. *J Continuing Educ Nurs* **271**: 17–27

Department of Health (1993) *A Vision for the Future. The Nursing Midwifery and Health Visiting Contribution to Health and Healthcare.* HMSO, London

Department of Health (1994) *Chief Nurse Officer Professional Letter.* **94**(5) HMSO, London

Dimond B (1995) *Legal Aspects of Nursing.* 2nd edn, Prentice Hall, Hemel Hempstead

Farrington A (1996) Clinical supervision: UKCC must be more proactive. *Br J Nurs* **512**: 716

Faugier J, Butterworth T (1994) *Clinical Supervision: A position paper.* School of Health Studies, University of Manchester, Manchester

Forchuk C (1993) *Hildegard E Peplau — Interpersonal Nursing Theory.* Sage Publications, London

Ford M, Walsh P (1995) *New Rituals for Old.* Butterworth-Heinmann Ltd, Oxford

Ghaye T, ed. (1996) *Creating Cultures for Improvement: Dialogues, Decisions and Dilemmas, CARN Critical Conversations: A Trilogy.* Hyde Publications, Bournemouth

Ghaye T *et al* (1996) *Professional Values: Being a Professional, Self-supported Learning Experiences for Healthcare Professionals.* Pentaxion Press, Newcastle-upon-Tyne

Ghaye T, Lillyman S (1997) *Learning Journals and Critical Incidents: Reflective Practice for Health Care Professionals.* Quay Books, Mark Allen Publishing, Salisbury

Ghaye T, Wakefield P eds (1993) *The Role of Self in Action Research, CARN Critical Conversations: A Trilogy.* Hyde Publications, Bournemouth

Kaberry S (1992) Supervision — support for nurses? *Senior Nurse* **12** (5): 24

Kohner N (1994) *Clinical Supervision in Practice.* Kings Fund Centre, London

Morgan C, Hughes R (1996) How can supervision become a real vision for the future? *J Psychiatr Mental Nurs* **3**: 117–24

Nicklin P (1995) Super supervision. *Nurs Management* **12** (5): 39

Peplau H (1988) *Interpersonal Relations in Nursing.* Macmillan, London

Plummer G, Edwards G, eds (1993) *Dimensions of action research: People, Practice and Power, CARN Critical Conversations: A Trilogy.* Hyde Publications, Bournemouth

Proctor B (1991) On being a trainer: Training and Supervision for Counselling in Action. in Hawkins B, Shoet R, eds, *Supervision in the helping professions.* Open University Press, Milton Keynes

Street A (1991) From Image to Action Reflection in Nursing Practice. in Palmer A *et al* (1994) *Reflective Practice in Nursing — The Growth of the Professional Practitioner.* Blackwell Science, Oxford: 2

United Kingdom Central Council for Nursing, Midwifery and Health Visiting (1992) *Code of Professional Conduct for the Nurse, Midwife and Health Visitor.* UKCC, London

United Kingdom Central Council for Nursing, Midwifery and Health Visiting (1996) *Position Statement on Clinical Supervision for Nursing and Health Visiting.* UKCC, London

Wright S (1989) *Changing Nursing Practice.* Arnold, London

Wright S (1997) Modelling excellence: the role of the consultant nurse. in *Clinical Supervision and Mentorship in Nursing.* Butterworth T, Faugier J, eds, Chapman and Hall, London

3

Some reflections on the implementation of clinical supervision

Gail Parsons

The UKCC (1996) claims that links between reflection and clinical supervision are the key to the development of professional nursing. With this in mind, the Dudley Group of Hospitals NHS Trust implemented a process of clinical supervision. The aims of this project were to improve practice, to meet new challenges effectively, and to implement changes in order to improve patient care and benefit care providers.

A steering group was formed, to include the nursing director and directorate nurse managers from a surgery and an orthopaedic ward. These two areas were chosen as pilot areas prior to introducing the process into the rest of the Trust. The focus of this process was on the E grade staff nurses who had a wealth of experience in their chosen specialities and who, to date, had no formal means of support in their place of work.

Getting started

Some of the key processes for introducing clinical supervision within the Trust included:

- awareness seminars for the implementation of clinical supervision for nurse managers and ward managers within the surgical and orthopaedic directorates
- consulting the target group (E grade staff nurses) to determine their 'readiness' for engaging in such an innovation
- attendance at a clinical supervision training course for the project leaders (three days)
- planning and delivering an in-house training programme for supervisors/supervisees.

The whole process would be monitored and evaluated. Recommendations for implementing clinical supervision Trust-wide would then be contained in a written report. I felt it was important to acknowledge that introducing clinical supervision would be a major change process (Kotter, 1996). Before its onset, a careful assessment had to be performed to discover the readiness of staff to participate in the project (Lancaster and Lancaster, 1982). This was identified in the staff consultations described above. I remember thinking: 'what a challenge!'

What does clinical supervision mean?

It was important that we had a clear understanding of the process of supervision and, in turn, shared our conceptions with others. My personal definition of what the term 'clinical supervision' means is: 'a support system which allows practitioners to form a professional, trusting relationship that enables them to reflect on their practice, to challenge the process, and then to move forward with improved knowledge and skills always aware of the impact of this from one's own professional values.' To complement this, the UKCC position statement on clinical supervision for nursing and health visiting (1996) states that clinical supervision is:

> *a practice-focused professional relationship involving a practitioner reflecting on practice guided by a skilled supervisor.*

Butterworth (1994) identifies the different processes of supervision as being associated with 'formative, restorative and normative' functions. The formative function is associated with education and reflection on an individual's practice; restorative function is the provision of supportive help for professionals working in a stressful and emotional environment; and the normative function considers the aspects of quality and leadership related to clinical practice.

Reflective conversations

The general feeling of ward managers and staff was congruent with the experience of others regarding the term 'clinical supervision'. 'Supervision' was seen as an inappropriate term, particularly as the group was seeing what was labelled 'clinical supervision' as a learning and enabling process. When discussing the process in some detail, we came to understand that our learning had to be made as visible as possible. The tacit and unconscious knowing had to be made more conscious and therefore more open to inspection and critique. We agreed that as nurses we should systematically record what we had learnt from our experiences (Benner, 1984). We discussed issues of confidentiality, record-keeping and the style and format of the 'learning record'. We appreciated that opinion is divided with regard to any kind of record of clinical supervision meetings being kept. We felt comfortable with the fact that a record would only be kept if both parties wanted it. We also reminded ourselves that the content of a record was a focus on individual and collective learning. Such a record would be kept by both the supervisor and the supervisee, and only they would have a right to divulge its contents to others.

The notion of the reflective conversation, as identified by Ghaye in *Chapter 4*, was used. The reflective conversation between the supervisor and the supervisee addressed particular 'points' which would act as an enabling framework for both parties. Nash (1996) indicates that communication should be central to the work of a profession that depends on interpersonal skills as much as on clinical skills. As a group we came to an understanding that reflective conversation lay at the heart of the clinical supervision process. Reflective conversation with peers was found to encourage the individual to analyse his or her own practice experiences and to help towards expanding personal knowledge in relation to nursing practice (Cowe, 1998). During the in-house training programme we practised this and group members expressed themselves openly. Their comments included: 'It almost felt false to begin with — this was due to the fact that I had known this nurse for eight years' and 'It could have easily developed into a chat if we had not used the framework as a guide.' The framework referred to, and identified by Ghaye in *Chapter 4*, was introduced to us by the in-house programme facilitator. It contains the following elements:

- a focus on caring values
- an appropriate question-and-answer-form
- looks back to what has been
- makes sense of practice through constructive challenge
- looks forward to what will or might be
- is a creative experience.

These elements were developed inductively from the facilitator's own work in clinical supervision with a variety of healthcare and education professionals. The framework provided 'signposts' for the participants which enabled them to discuss clinical, managerial and other issues. The structure is merely a facilitating framework, not an enslaving one to be assiduously worked right through during each session. We felt it gave our conversations a sense of purpose and direction.

There was a consensus of opinion regarding the unavoidable difficulty of 'changing the course of the conversation' if a supervisee wished to discuss his or her personal issues at the planned session. This difficulty was carefully discussed and it was agreed that certain professional and personal matters are closely linked. If professional issues are addressed and personal issues are ignored, it may cause the relationship between the two professionals to become 'strained' or even to break down (Goorapah, 1997). However, we felt it was important for the participants to ensure that ground rules were set before the process began. These 'rules' incorporated the following ideals: confidentiality, autonomy, self-disclosure, no put-downs, commitment and reciprocity (Bond and Holland, 1998). The issue: 'How does one end a supervision session?' also arose. Time is a finite resource and the framework allows for appropriate closure to take place. A rounding-up of the major things learned and, where appropriate, some action planning can form the closing phase.

In-house supervisors'/supervisees' training

Information packages and pre-course reading lists were issued to the participants prior to a one-day training session. The aim of the training was to equip all members of staff to try to begin to undertake clinical supervision within their workplace. The content of the training addressed a number of questions and covered a variety of processes, including:

- exploring conceptions of clinical supervision
- practising holding truly reflective conversations
- discussing how to move clinical supervision forward
- discussing how to keep it going — sustainability
- discussing how we know if it is working — evaluation.

In particular, the focus on our 'caring values' — making sense of clinical action and its potential to enlighten and empower — was identified during the training day.

Evaluation of the project

An evaluation day was held for all the participants of the project. The course evaluation that we undertook was illuminating and generally positive, with every member feeling able to return to their workplace and try to implement clinical supervision. Some of the major things we learned were to do with developing a shared view of clinical supervision, trying to make quality time available and the way the culture of the clinical environment influenced both the clinical supervision implementation process and what was discussed in supervision sessions. For example:

1 The participants of the project thought that other staff
   needed an understanding of what clinical supervision was so
   that there was a shared understanding within the workplace.
   This would be helpful not only for other trained staff but
   also for nursing auxiliaries and student nurses.
2 It had been difficult to avoid interruptions during some
   supervision sessions, as private space within the hospital
   environment was difficult to find. One supervisor
   commented:

   *I was carrying the hospital bleep and had planned a
   supervision session for the afternoon. Unfortunately there
   was no one who could take the bleep from me, and I did not
   want to cancel because of this. We were interrupted three
   times, which was really annoying as we were discussing
   important issues.*

   Another member of staff said:

   *I looked forward to my one-hour session, and when asked
   by a member of staff where could I be contacted if I was
   needed, I was inclined not to tell in case I was called back!
   After all, I had some important points to discuss with my
   supervisor.*

3 We began to appreciate that implementing effective clinical
   supervision was as much about workplace culture as it was

about working closely with staff, helping and supporting them to take practice forward.

The Work Environment Scale (WES) questionnaire

The importance of workplace culture in implementing effective clinical supervision was vividly highlighted by the results of a WES (Moos, 1994) questionnaire customised for the group by the in-house facilitator. Data from the questionnaire was used to make graphs of nurses' perceptions of the culture of their clinical environments. The data enable individual and nurse group perceptions to be compared meaningfully. The graphs illustrate three important dimensions that make up the workplace environment or culture. They are to do with personal growth, interpersonal relationships and the way the 'system' maintains or changes itself. Within each dimension there are a number of sub-scales.

Due to issues of confidentiality, I cannot present the data in any detail here. What I can do is to present two descriptive portraits that summarise some of the data about nurse perceptions of workplace culture in two different clinical areas. I will then go on to discuss some of the 'big messages' that emerged about the implementation of clinical supervision and which are likely to be transferable to other Trusts.

Portrait one

The major attributes of the culture here are the very low levels of line manager support (the extent to which management is supportive of nurses and encourages nurses to be supportive of one another) and 'physical comfort' coupled with very high 'work pressure' (the extent to which high work demands and time pressure dominate the work milieu). Also, the data shows relatively low scores in relation to perceptions of 'autonomy' (how much the nurses are encouraged to be self-sufficient and make their own decisions) and 'clarity' (whether the nurses know what to expect in their daily routine and how explicitly rules and policies are communicated). Nursing staff in this clinical environment who completed the WES questionnaire, were aware of the need for good planning, efficiency and getting the job done ('task orientation'). There is a suggestion in the data that they do this by being friendly and supportive of each other ('co-worker cohesion'). There are some clear indications here of specific 'work stressors' and some coping responses.

Portrait two

The major attributes of the workplace culture here are high levels of 'involvement' (this is about nurses' levels of concern and commitment to their jobs), 'co-worker cohesion', 'control' (management's use of rules and procedures in practice) and 'innovation' (the emphasis on variety, change and new approaches). The level of line manager support is high. The scores for 'autonomy' are average but this is not surprising given the emphasis on teamwork evident from the other scores. Scores for 'physical comfort' (the extent to which the physical surroundings contribute to a pleasant work environment) are relatively low.

So what can we learn from this?

In the context of implementing and sustaining clinical supervision, the results from the WES questionnaire tell us a number of things:

1   The data from the questionnaire highlighted differences
    between these two clinical areas. In one there appears to be a
    strong sense of teamwork and team spirit, with nurses and
    management working supportively with each other. This
    seems to help offset work pressures and create a culture of
    planned innovation. Data from the other clinical area present
    much food for thought. They exhibit some of the
    characteristics of a disempowering and 'challenging' clinical
    environment, and the ingredients for a lowering of nurse
    morale, for stress, burnout and occupational disenchantment.
2   The data can be presented in an understandable form and
    used by the supervisor and supervisee in a catalytic manner
    to help focus their reflective conversations on such issues as
    personal growth, on issues to do with self and others and on
    issues about how these relate to working effectively and
    competently in the 'system'.
3   The data suggested to us that the likelihood of clinical
    supervision 'taking a grip' and becoming embedded as part
    of professional practice, is likely to depend on perceived
    levels of 'work pressure', management 'support', individual

'involvement' and the existence of an 'innovatory climate'. One of the clinical areas seems much better placed than the other in these respects.

4   The process of clinical supervision in facilitating the personal growth of healthcare professionals, in developing effective teams and in enhancing work in a clinical area, cannot be assumed to be unproblematic. It is likely to be a bumpy process.

To conclude

All of this has helped us to develop two important insights. Firstly, that simply 'delivering' the same clinical supervision training to healthcare professionals from different clinical areas is in itself no guarantee, either of its workplace relevance or of its usefulness to the individuals. Secondly, that we might usefully rethink the content of such training. We might, perhaps, pay relatively less attention to the interpersonal skills dimension and more time developing nurses' political acuity. Clinical supervision operates in a context. We have learnt that it is important to come to know this context. Some contexts are more supportive while others are much less receptive to initiatives such as clinical supervision. Reflection on our actions has made us all more aware of the personal, professional and political aspects of trying to implement clinical supervision.

References

Benner P (1984) *From Novice To Expert.* Addison-Wesley, California

Bond M, Holland S (1998) *Skills of Clinical Supervision for Nurses.* Open University Press, Milton Keynes

Butterworth T (1994) Preparing to take on Clinical Supervision. *Nurs Stand* **21**(8): 32–4

Cowe F (1998) Clinical Supervision for Specialist Nurses. *Professional Nurse* **13**(5): 284–7

Goorapah D (1997) Review article: Clinical Supervision. *J Clin Nurs* **6**: 173–8

Kotter J (1996) *Leading Change.* Harvard Business School Press, USA: 9

Lancaster J, Lancaster W (1982) *Concepts for Advanced Nursing Practice. The Nurse as a Change Agent.* CV Mosby Company, London: 22

Moos R (1994) *The Work Environment Scale.* Consulting Psychologists Press Inc., California

Nash J (1996) The Route to Effective Nurse–Patient Communication. *Nurs Times* **92**(17)

Nazarko L (1997) A Few Home Truths. *Nurs Times* **93**(39): 75–6

United Kingdom Central Council (1996) *Position Statement on Clinical Supervision for Nursing and Health Visiting.* UKCC, London

4
The role of reflection in nurturing creative clinical conversations

Tony Ghaye

Healthcare professionals have many different roles. Every day they may juggle clinical, professional, managerial and research roles. They also perform numerous tasks which may be variously regarded as 'basic' or 'routine', 'ordinary' or 'extraordinary', 'special' or 'enjoyable', and so on. In all of this — whether it is when washing an elderly patient, combing a woman's hair and deciding whether or not to put in her rollers, trying to explain to a student nurse that her manner is somewhat abrasive, trying to relate meaningfully to a patient suffering from a chronic form of dementia, or breaking the news of a healthy newborn baby to an expectant family, and much, much more — we need to be particularly conscious of the power of language. When we are being the patient's advocate we are, in an important sense, enabling the patient to have a voice; enabling his or her thoughts, emotions, hopes and anxieties to find expression. Each one of us has a voice, although it may of course be expressed in very different ways. With this thought in mind, I suggest that two fundamental skills necessary for all healthcare professionals are firstly, to discover and reflect on their own voice and secondly, to enable others to hear and claim their own.

In the context of this book, the idea of voice finds expression and significance in a particular kind of dialogue which a supervisor and a supervisee might have when engaging in the learning process called 'clinical supervision'. I am going to call this type of dialogue 'a reflective conversation'. In doing so, I am suggesting two things. Firstly, that the interactive dialogue of supervision may usefully be described as conversational and, secondly, that in order for clinical supervision to be about learning, this conversation needs to be reflective in kind. By implication, then, I am saying that reflective conversation is at the very heart of the clinical supervision process. In this chapter, I shall briefly set out Schon's original view (1983) of a reflective conversation — one which is described in greater detail in Ghaye and Lillyman (2000) — and then I shall show how I have extended and reconstructed Schon's original view so that we might gain a sense of the role of reflection in nurturing a creative clinical conversation.

A reflective conversation with a situation: the work of Schon

Schon has made an important contribution to our understanding of reflective practices. In his book, *The Reflective Practitioner* (1983), we find a number of key ideas which have subsequently been applied to healthcare and woven into a series of texts designed to enhance the practice of healthcare professionals (see for example, Ghaye and Lillyman, 2000; Ghaye, Gillespie and Lillyman, 2000). Central to Schon's argument are ideas related to what we know and how this 'knowing' is put into action. He argues that much of this 'knowing' is hard to put into words (Schon, 1987). The 'knowing' is very often described as 'unconscious', 'tacit' (Polanyi, 1958), and even as 'unarticulated commonsense'. It does, however, reveal itself in our actions; in other words, in what we do when caring for others. In saying this, Schon is raising a number of important and problematic issues. Firstly, and by implication, he is helping us to appreciate that professional healthcare knowledge is describable, can be seen in action, can be understood by others and, therefore, can be opened up to inquiry and public scrutiny. This body of knowledge, then, is a source of professional accountability. Secondly, Schon is suggesting that we might usefully reflect on our 'knowing- in-action'; in order to improve what we do, we should reflect on our practice. In terms of healthcare, this might be reflecting on some puzzling, troubling, interesting, promising or surprising phenomenon with which we are trying to deal. There are two parts to this important idea of his. This process might take place in the heat of the moment, when we have to think on our feet, and is described by Schon as 'reflection-in-action'. Alternatively, the reflection might take place later, out of the clinical area, and thus be described as 'reflection-on-action'. Thirdly, Schon describes a process of improvement whereby, literally through conversation, situations which are uncertain, unstable, unique and value-laden come to be known, better understood, handled and managed. The process is not unlike the sort of thing that might take place in many clinical supervision meetings. For example, after the initial presentation of the topic of conversation — what Schon calls 'the framing of the problem' — there is a:

> *web of moves, consequences, implications, appreciations*
> *and further moves... some moves are resisted while others*
> *generate new phenomena.*

(Schon, 1983, p.94).

Through this conversation with the situation, the participants have to:

> *listen to the situation's back-talk, forming new appre-*
> *ciations which guide further moves.*

(p.94)

This is an interactive process of construction and reconstruction of meanings and actions. Schon called it 'framing and reframing the problem'. It is both energised and made possible through a reflective conversation with a situation. But the process is not an easy one. In being open to the 'situation's back-talk', the participant:

> *must be willing to enter into new confusions and*
> *uncertainties. Hence, he must adopt a kind of double*
> *vision. He must act in accordance with the view he has*
> *adopted, but he must recognise that he can always break it*
> *open later, indeed, must break it open later in order to*
> *make new sense of his transaction with the situation. This*
> *becomes more difficult to do as the process continues. His*
> *choices become more committing; his moves, more nearly*
> *irreversible. As the risk of uncertainty increases, so does*
> *the temptation to treat the view as the reality.*

(p.164)

The first message here is that improving our thinking, practice and the context in which our healthcare work is embedded, needs to be seen as a continuous and lifelong learning process. The second message is more contentious. To say that as the process unfurls and the conversation develops, choices become more committing and irreversible is to devalue and deny the power that certain kinds of reflection and reflective practices have to guard against this very thing. In summary, then, Schon describes reflective practice as taking the form of a 'reflective conversation with the situation' between two people. He makes a clear distinction between the reflective practitioner and the client, with the former facilitating the conversation. The interaction between the two is conditioned by something called a 'reflective contract' where the two agree to:

> *enquire into the situation, for which the client seeks help;*

> *to try to understand what he is experiencing and to make*
> *that understanding accessible to the practitioner when he*
> *does not understand or agree... . The practitioner agrees*
> *to deliver competent performance to the limits of his*
> *capacity; to help the client understand the meaning of the*
> *professional's advice and the rationale for his actions,*
> *while at the same time he tries to learn the meanings his*
> *actions have for his client; to make himself readily con-*
> *frontable by his client; and to reflect on his own tacit*
> *understandings when he needs to do so in order to play his*
> *part in fulfilling the contract.*
>
> (Schon, 1983, p.27)

The notion of a reflective contract is, in essence, a helpful one in the context of clinical supervision, but not without its problems. Briefly, and on the positive side, the idea of some kind of 'contract' or agreement between the participants might be very useful as it symbolises the importance of the process, can help to delineate roles and responsibilities and clarify what might usefully be expected in terms of processes and outcomes of the supervisory meetings. In his paper about a palliative model of clinical supervision, Jones (1997) alludes to what might form the content and process of such an agreement; an agreement that manifests itself as 'an experiential infrastructure' (p.1029). On the cautionary side, the formulation of any kind of reflective contract requires careful consideration of the nature of (and demands on) competence, criteria for satisfaction, issues of power and gender, a host of ethical issues to do with record keeping, confidentiality and codes of practice, as well as knowing how to handle feelings of anger, compliancy, resentment, dis-illusionment and success. All of these things need to be carefully thought through.

Clinical supervision and the creation of knowledge to improve practice

In this chapter I am going to argue, as others have done (Kohner, 1994), that reflection on practice is the central component of clinical supervision. Reflections of one kind or another and the ways we use them are, collectively, the enabling process by and through which the participants learn together. Clinical supervision therefore embraces three types of action:

- **committed action** where the participants have a strong sense of commitment to learn — through conversation, from experience — and to enquire into practice
- **intentional action** where the participants seek to reflect systematically, critically and creatively on practice with the intention of improving thinking, practice and clinical area in some way
- **informed action** which stems from sustained reflective conversations that enable the participants to be clear about their own motives and professional values, and how both of these guide and shape clinical action.

I am also asserting that the reflective conversation is about healthcare professionals seeking their own voice; an authentic voice and one that enables them to talk about their experiences and their ability — or not — to learn from the work that they do. As in any conversation that takes place in an appropriate setting and with respected and respectful 'others', clinical supervision is an opportunity for the healthcare professional to speak out, to ask questions, to challenge, to contest conventions and routines, and to imagine and enact creative and ethical ways to enhance the quality of the care they are able to give. In essence, then, clinical supervision is about developing our practice through a richer and more holistic appreciation of it. It is a process of thinking in conversation with others. It is also a process of knowledge creation which challenges the still (alas) pervasive notion in healthcare of technical rationality (Schon, 1983). In this way it decentralises the production of healthcare knowledge, removing it from being the monopoly of universities, governments and research centres separated from the world of practice, from whence it is handed down and magically applied to the everyday problems of clinical work. The reflective clinical conversation is a process through which healthcare practitioners create their own practical and living theories which serve to guide and explain their everyday practice. In this way they do not just 'use' someone else's theories but create their own by engaging in an ongoing conversation about the meaning and consequences of their experience and actions, and the historical contexts, social structures and political processes which serve to liberate, constrain or distort their ability to think and act creatively, competently and ethically (Ghaye *et al*, 1996; Whitehead, 1993; Winter, 1998).

The reflective clinical conversation

The role and nature of a reflective clinical conversation has, in my view, been underemphasised in the clinical supervision literature. This, I believe, stems from three kinds of debilitating beliefs. The first is the debilitating 'toolbox' mentality. When we are in this frame of mind we reduce the preparation for and processes of clinical supervision to the acquisition of a set of skills rather than an entire approach to professional practice. At its worst, reflection becomes yet another skill such as active listening — the ability to empathise and to conduct appropriate questioning. Reflection then joins an ever-lengthening list of 'skills for effective supervision'. Fish and Twinn (1997) present a cogent argument supporting the view that clinical supervision should be part of the big picture of developing one's professionality, and not just a set of skills or competencies.

The second debilitating belief is that reflection is some kind of flat, unproblematic, uni-dimensional idea that we can confidently use in the singular. There are, in fact, many kinds of reflection which serve different interests and purposes (Ghaye and Lillyman, 1997).

The idea that professional practice is about the transmission and application of knowledge to known situations in order to produce rational solutions to pre-specified problems, is the third and final debilitating belief (Lester, 1995). In tomorrow's health service, the competent and confident practitioners will be those who are able continually to reconstruct and evolve their practice. This will be a creative process fuelled by reflections on experience. The reflective conversation will therefore be an opportunity to develop creative and situationally relevant, value-based ethical understandings that have the potential to meet constantly changing healthcare challenges and situations (The Open University, 1998).

Over the past five years in my work with practitioners engaged in various English National Board courses, university award-bearing degree programmes with a reflective practice dimension, and a variety of study days and network meetings on clinical supervision, I have been able to distil what might be regarded as some of the most important characteristics or qualities of a reflective clinical conversation. My curiosity has been stimulated by three questions:

1 So, what is a reflective conversation?
2 How far would I recognise one if I heard one?
3 How would I set about facilitating and nurturing a
  conversation of this kind?

Qualities of the reflective clinical conversation

Has a focus on caring values

In order for a dialogue to be termed a 'reflective conversation', there needs to be some consideration and questioning of the caring values that the healthcare professionals are committed to, and try to live out in their work. Professional and personal values are those fundamentally important things that make healthcare professionals the kind of people they are; they give their caring work its shape, form and purpose. Coming to know them, justifying and living them out is something to which it is worthy to aspire. None of this is easy, though. Even quite experienced practitioners have difficulties in articulating their values and addressing those things that get in the way of putting values into practice (Ghaye *et al*, 1996b). To act confidently, competently and creatively we need to reflect on our caring intentions, the ends we have in mind and the means we might choose in order to achieve them. The reflective conversation is the medium through which we are able to do this. The focus on values is a fundamental characteristic of a conversation of this kind. It is one where practitioners interrogate, question and reinterpret the values that guide what they do in the context in which they find themselves working. Without this focus on values, I suggest the conversation is not truly reflective, but something else — a conversation that is more technically focused, for example. Just as some argue that not all thinking about practice is reflective if there is no questioning of goals and values (Zeichner and Liston, 1996), I would argue that a reflective conversation about means and healthcare ends is not reflective if it does not involve a discussion about values. A focus on values gives the supervisee the opportunity to reveal joys and achievements as values are lived out in practice. Such a focus may also expose the frustrations and contradictions in caring work when values are negated in practice.

Takes an appropriate question-and-answer form

If learning through clinical supervision is about learning through conversation, then it is important for the participants to have a repertoire of questions that enable them to gain some critical distance from their work in order to confront aspects of it and come to know it differently. Such questions can be of many kinds (Smyth, 1991), but four fundamental questions are:

1 What is my practice like?
2 Why is it like this?
3 How has it come to be this way?
4 What would I like to improve, how and why?

These are challenging questions indeed. Other relevant ones might be:

- How far do I live my caring values out in my work?
- Whose interests are served or denied by my/our practice?
- What organisational and other influences prevent me/us working in alternative ways?
- Indeed, what alternatives are available?

There are a great many reflective questions (Tomm, 1987). The method of conversational analysis that is described in the book, *Reflection: Principles and practice for healthcare professionals* (Ghaye and Lillyman, 2000), calls different reflective questions 'leads'; the supervisee's responses of one kind or another are called 'reflections' and the various ways the supervisor and supervisee sustain and develop the conversation are called 'connections'. In that book I draw upon the transcript of one clinical supervision meeting to show how we might answer questions of the following kind:

1 How far can the dialogue between supervisor and supervisee be described as a conversation?
2 How far is it a reflective and creative conversation?
3 What is the evidence to support or refute questions 1 and 2?
4 So what might we learn from using this method of conversational analysis?

The skill of nurturing a reflective conversation is linked to knowing just what to ask, when and in what way. Even more important, for some clinical conversations, is to know just when to stop asking questions, to do other things and to enable the silence to be seen as a potentially rich, creative space. This is the type of sensitivity that is not easily 'taught' on courses that purport to prepare healthcare workers for clinical supervision. Which of our verbal contributions, our listening and thinking contributions are most helpful when the supervisee feels that he or she is 'stuck' or in a 'stand-still' situation (Andersen, 1991)? In addition, nurturing reflective conversation is about understanding the complexity of human communication and information processing. For example:

> ... *human communication is a complex interactive process*

in which meanings are generated, maintained and/or changed through recursive interaction between human beings. Communication is not to be taken as a simple linear process of transmitting messages from an active sender to a passive receiver; rather, it is a circular, interactive process of co-creation by the participants involved.

(Poskiparta, Kettunen and Liimatainen, 1998, p.683)

Is located in time and space

The reflective conversation is an artefact of the moment. It is located in time, has antecedents and consequences. In this sense it has an historical dimension. Its co-construction occupies a socio-political space, too. What is disclosed in a clinical supervision meeting is therefore subject to these and other influences. Space also has a geographical expression, so finding a comfortable room or an area where a conversation can be developed is fundamental. To value reflective conversations appropriately, they need to be seen as part of an extended dialogue between supervisor and supervisee, recorded in some mutually acceptable manner, reflected upon and compared over time. In this way recurring patterns of interest and concern have the chance to emerge. When these are visible and more fully known we may have increased options for action and/or acquire insights that might enable us to think differently.

Looks back to what has been

This is probably the most widely accepted view of reflection and one that describes it as an essentially retrospective activity, but there is a lot more to reflection than this. A commitment to look back is also a commitment to adopt a 'reflective posture'. This idea comes from the work of Freire (1972). He described the hallmarks of this posture as conversationalists examining their experience critically, questioning and interpreting it and doing this in public and not in isolation from others. Three important factors emerge here. Firstly, in clinical supervision the 'raw material', so to speak, is previous experience. It is this that fuels and energises the reflective processes. Secondly, a commitment to a reflective posture has to be understood to be a shared responsibility between supervisor and supervisee. And finally, this expression of reflection is not the commonly held one that equates it with some kind of solitary, introspective and private activity. Moreover, it is a view of reflection that is more collaborative, public and discursive in nature.

Makes sense of caring work through constructive challenge

Healthcare professionals have to make sense of their work in the context in which it occurs. They have to make sense of the perceived and actual impact of their caring work on their clients, the families and on their colleagues. In reflective clinical conversations the important goal is to try to achieve a greater sense of clarity and certainty that practice can become even more clinically effective, professional and ethical. Moving practice forward is stifled if this sense-making quality of the clinical conversation is absent. It is, however, a complex and potentially uncomfortable process, and one that is dependent upon a shared commitment from the participants to challenge and confront practice. To move forward implies that we have a greater sense of self and professional identity in relation to practice. In the post-modern and de-traditionalising society described by Glenn (1999):

> *the requirement to construct a personal and professional self, as a continuing process, becomes more acutely necessary than ever before... . To have a self was to be someone of a particular sort; now however, to have a self is to discover who one is through what one does.*
>
> (pp.5–6)

Making sense of self through reflections on practice needs to be viewed as an active, challenging and creative process of jointly constructed interpretations (Newman and Holzman, 1997).

Looks forward to what will or might be

Taylor (1989, p.47) suggests that, 'in order to have a sense of who we are, we have to have a notion of how we have become and where we are going'. Reflection is not only concerned with looking back but also with looking into the future; with where we are going. Working with experience is the key here. Centrally, the reflective clinical conversation is about acknowledging the importance of working with experience. In acknowledging this we should be cautious about simply giving primacy to experience without taking into account the context in which, and through which, the experience has come about. Clinical experience should not be celebrated uncritically. Simply having experiences to recount in a clinical supervision meeting does not necessarily mean that they are reflected upon in the way I am suggesting in this chapter. The clinical supervision meeting should be a context, or facilitating framework, for learning. All such frameworks contain 'taken-for-granted assumptions about what it is legitimate to do, to say and even think' (Boud and Miller, 1996, p.18). Through conversations of the kind I am suggesting, looking into the future provides an opportunity to think creatively. Being creative opens up possibilities and avenues for new and improved action.

Has the potential to enlighten and empower

If the clinical conversation is truly reflective, it can also be called creative. The creative conversation can be linked to notions of enlightenment and empowerment. This is the subject of another book in this series (Ghaye, Gillespie and Lillyman, 2000). In brief, the creative clinical conversation is a process whereby we try to add meaning and value to what the practitioner claims to know and do. This reconstructed and refocused practice can be described as more 'enlightened'. Reflective conversations that are empowering enable healthcare workers to name, to define and to construct their own 'realities', to gain a greater sense of control over their professional lives and to develop more authentic selves. However:

> *... it must also be asked whether organisations want an empowered workforce. Indeed to suggest reflection as a process of empowerment suggests that nurses have to assert self against power gradients of more powerful others, whose own interests may be compromised. Nurses may have internalised a sense of the powerless self through working in bureaucratic settings which have taught everyone to be compliant, to be rule governed, and not to ask questions, seek alternatives or deal with competing values.*

> (Johns, 1998, p.12)

Perhaps the best way to try to improve practice lies not so much in trying to control people's behaviours, as in helping them to control their own by becoming more aware of what they are doing (Elliott, 1987).

Evidence-based practice and the reflective clinical conversation

The reflective clinical conversation touches on many contemporary political and professional initiatives designed to both modernise and improve the quality of patient care. It can also be related to what might be regarded as the essence of good caring practice. For example, in *A First Class Service* (NHS Executive, 1998), the government sets out its plans to improve the NHS. The three central elements here are professional self-regulation, clinical governance and lifelong learning. In important ways the reflective clinical conversation makes a contribution to each of these elements. Reflection, both in-action and on-practice, that is undertaken in a systematic, sustained, public and constructively critical manner, is a process of individual and collective regulation. It is also about self and group regeneration. This regeneration is linked to the idea that healthcare can, in very significant ways, be 'transformed' through reflective practices (Johns and Freshwater, 1998). A commitment to become a reflective practitioner should be a wholehearted and sincere one, for we cannot be reflective practitioners one day and something else another. Reflective practitioners appreciate that learning is a continuous interplay between action and reflections on it. They have a commitment to the principle of lifelong learning. In Ghaye and Lillyman (2000) we have also said that reflection should have a consequence. This consequence is that it should strive to improve thinking and practice and the context in which these take place. Reflective practices are supportive of, and also contribute towards, initiatives for improved clinical effectiveness. If clinical governance is 'the process by which each part of the NHS quality assures its clinical decisions' (NHS Executive, 1998), then some kind of synergy between this and reflective practices needs to be made.

It goes without saying that practice development must surely have 'a firm evidential base' (Walsh, 1999). It must be grounded in it and see evidence as its friend, for it is essentially about the process of improvement. So, where might we derive such evidence? Reflective practices are an important source for they are evidence-based. Reflection is not simply a private, solitary, navel-gazing activity where we replay and rehearse in the comfort of an armchair some of the things we have recently encountered in our work. Although, for some, reflection might have elements of privacy and solitude about it, we should not forget that reflection also has a public and political face. Practice development, or we might call it 'practice improvement', is a technical, professional and political activity. It is also essentially judgmental in that we have to make decisions about preferred courses of action, and judgements about what might count as 'a development' or 'an improvement'. In the context of clinical supervision all sorts of improvements can be sensed, explored and tested out. If an agreement can be reached about the need to record the supervision meeting in some appropriate way, the record can become an important source of evidence; the catalyst if you like, for further conversations which have the potential to take practice forward. *Table 4.1* (on *page 69*) is a simple form based on the qualities of the reflective clinical conversation set out in this chapter. It has been used by healthcare practitioners to do three things:

1 To add some kind of structure to the clinical conversation. It shows the participants the kind of topics that are likely to be talked about. Some may be discussed more than others. The sheet also addresses the issue of expectation. Both the supervisor and supervisee know, in advance, the territory that will, or might be explored.
2 To record evidence of how the participants engaged with each of the elements of the reflective conversation. These can be words, key phrases or short sentences.
3 To provide evidence towards the end of the meeting to review the ground that has been covered, the ways in which it has been covered, and as a springboard to discuss what might happen next.

Supervisors may find the form useful in the way it illuminates the difference between the qualities the conversation did have, ought to or might have had. The supervisee might have talked a great deal about 'what has been' and spent relatively little time on 'what will or might be'. There may of course be good reasons for this. However, both parties might come to appreciate that two of the reasons were that there was little or no evidence recorded in the boxes labelled 'making sense of practice through constructive challenge' and 'caring values in action'. This kind of review can therefore help the participants to get the most out of their meeting, can provide clues about how useful the meeting was and can identify the ragged edges, messy bits and unfinished business.

In conclusion

To conclude, I want to pencil in two important connections. Earlier I suggested that the reflective clinical conversation could be related to the essence of what might be regarded as good caring practice. For example, Campbell (1984) described the nurse as a 'skilled companion', to 'be with the patient' and 'doing things for them'. We can draw a connection here with the role of the supervisor as a skilled companion of the supervisee, being with them and enabling them to think through improvements to their practice. Secondly, Kitson (1999) talks about the importance of the person as a fundamental element of nursing and how this is enshrined in nursing's practical and intellectual history. Drawing on her earlier work (Kitson, 1998) and that of MacIntyre (1985) she states:

> *The first essence or essential element in nursing is the philosophical and moral recognition of nursing as a person-centred activity. With this acknowledgement comes a set of beliefs and values... about the uniqueness of the individual, his or her needs and how he or she should be treated. Also comes along a set of attitudes and behaviours required for the nurse to operate in a person-centred way. Techniques include paying attention to detail, uncovering meaning in everyday situations, being attentive and available, reliable and true to promises, understanding the importance of each person's own particular biography and how he or she is seeking to gain an understanding of what is happening to him or her.*
>
> (p.44)

In an important and humanly significant way these espoused beliefs could also reflect much of the essence of the process of nurturing creative clinical conversations.

Table 4.1 Qualities of the reflective clinical conversation

Supervisor:		Supervisee:	Date:
Topic of conversation:			
Qualities of the conversation	Evidence		
1 *Has a focus on caring values*			
2 *Takes an appropriate question-and-answer form*			
3 *Looks back to what has been*			
4 *Makes sense of practice through constructive challenge*			
5 *Looks forward to what will or might be*			
6 *Is a creative experience*			
Action to be taken:	What?	By whom?	When?
Signed:	Supervisor:	Supervisee:	Next meeting:

References

Andersen T, ed. (1991) *The Reflecting Team: Dialogues and Dialogues about Dialogues.* W Norton and Company, New York

Boud D, Miller N (1996) *Working with Experience: Animating Learning.* Routledge, London

Campbell A (1984) Nursing, nurturing and sexism. in Campbell A, ed. *Moderated Love: A Theology of Professional Care.* SPCK, London

Elliott J (1987) Educational theory, practical philosophy and action research. *Br J Educational Studies,* **35**: 149–69

Fish D, Twinn S (1997) *Quality Clinical Supervision in the Health Care Professions.* Butterworth Heinnemann, Oxford

Freire P (1972) *Pedagogy of the Oppressed.* Penguin, Harmondsworth

Ghaye T, Gillespie D, Lillyman S, eds, (2000) *Empowerment Through Reflection: The narratives of healthcare professionals.* Quay Books, Mark Allen Publishing Group, Salisbury

Ghaye T, Lillyman S (1997) *Learning Journals and Critical Incidents: Reflective practice for healthcare professionals.* Quay Books, Mark Allen Publishing Group, Salisbury

Ghaye T, Lillyman S (2000) *Reflection: Principles and practice for healthcare professionals.* Quay Books, Mark Allen Publishing Group, Salibury

Ghaye T, Lillyman S, eds (2000) *Caring Moments: The discourse of reflective practice.* Quay Books, Mark Allen Publishing Group, Salisbury

Ghaye T, Cuthbert S, Danai K, *et al* (1996a) *Theory-Practice Relationships: Reconstructing Practice, Learning through Critical Reflective Practice, Self-Supported Learning Experiences for Healthcare Professionals.* Pentaxion Press, Newcastle upon Tyne

Ghaye T, Cuthbert S, Danai K *et al* (1996b) *Professional Values: Being a Professional, Learning through Critical Reflective Practice, Self-Supported Learning Experiences for Healthcare Professionals.* Pentaxion Press, Newcastle upon Tyne

Glen S (1999) Health Care Education for dialogue and dialogic relationships. *Nurs Ethics* **6** (1): 3–11

Johns C (1998) Opening the Doors of Perception. in Johns C, Freshwater D, eds, *Transforming Nursing through Reflective Practice.* Blackwell Science, Oxford

Johns C, Freshwater D, eds (1998) *Transforming Nursing through Reflective Practice.* Blackwell Science, Oxford

Jones A (1997) A 'bonding between strangers': a palliative model of clinical supervision. *J Adv Nurs* **26**: 1028–35

Kitson A (1999) The Essence of Nursing. *Nursing Standard,* **13** (23): 42–6

Kitson A (1998) *Whose death is it anyway? The Abbeyfield Lecture 1998.* Abbeyfield Society, St Albans

Kohner N (1994) *Clinical Supervision: An Executive Summary.* Kings Fund, London

Lester S (1995) Beyond Knowledge and Competence. *Capability* **1** (3) Higher Education Capability

MacIntyre A (1985) *After Virtue: A study in moral theory.* 2nd edn, Duckworth, London

Newman F, Holzman L (1997) *The End of Knowing: A new developmental way of knowing.* Routledge, London

NHS Executive (1998) *A First Class Service: Quality in the New NHS.* NHS Executive, Leeds

Polanyi M (1958), *Personal Knowledge.* Oxford University Press, Oxford

Poskiparta M, Kettunen T, Liimatainen L (1998) Reflective Questions in Health Counselling. *Qualitative Health Res* **8**(5): 682–93

Schon D (1983) *The Reflective Practitioner: How professionals think in action.* Basic Books, New York

Schon D (1987) *Educating the Reflective Practitioner.* Jossey Bass, London

Smyth J (1991) *Teachers as Collaborative Learners.* Open University Press, Milton Keynes

Taylor C (1989) *Sources of the Self.* Cambridge University Press, Cambridge

The Open University (1998) *K509 Clinical Supervision: A development pack for nurses.* The Open University, Milton Keynes

Tomm K (1987) Interventive Interviewing: Part II. Reflective questioning as a means to enable self-healing. *Fam Process* **26**: 167–83

Walsh M (1999) Nurses and Nurse practitioners, Part 2: Perspectives on Care. *Nursing Standard* **13**(25): 36–40

Whitehead J (1993) *The Growth of Educational Knowledge: Creating your own living educational theories.* Hyde Publications, Bournemouth

Winter R (1998) Finding a Voice: Thinking with others: a conception of action research. *Educational Action Research* **6**(1): 53–68

Zeichner K, Liston D (1996) *Reflective Teaching: An Introduction.* Lawrence Earlbaum Associates, New Jersey

5

Connecting reflective practice with clinical supervision

Dawn Pattison, Dorothy Parsons and Clare Weatherhead

Introduction

The value of clinical supervision and reflective practice has been highlighted in many key documents and in the nursing press. Successful implementation can lead to advancements of safe nursing practice and professional development. As senior nurses working in neighbouring critical care areas, we were and are keen to implement clinical supervision successfully within our clinical environments. The aim is to maintain and to improve standards of care whilst encouraging personal and professional reflection. The purpose of this chapter is to try to identify the points of contact between reflective practice and clinical supervision and how the latter can be successfully implemented within two similar emergency settings.

Most recent organisational restructuring within the Trust has included the opening of an emergency assessment unit that operates alongside the accident and emergency department, receiving acute medical referrals from general practitioners. The unit comprises a six-bedded area with, at present, six members of staff. There is no formal process of supervision within this area but senior staff are keen to initiate clinical supervision in order to safeguard standards of practice. Also, as the emergency assessment unit is unique to the hospital, the staff are keen to work with colleagues in accident and emergency, to talk through any problems or situations they come across. It is hoped that this process will facilitate the transference of knowledge and skills. It is also seen as collaborative working. Clinical supervision was introduced within accident and emergency in 1995 following a pilot study supported by our Trust. Accident and emergency was one of three areas within the hospital included in the pilot. One-to-one clinical supervision currently occurs there.

Some views of reflective practice

Reflective practices could be employed in order to discover what knowledge, skills and attitudes nurses employ, and to what extent they are applied. Popper (1965) proposed that knowledge of the world comes to each individual in various different ways, amongst these are perception and understanding. According to De Bono (1979) perception is the way we see the world, and we only notice things if we pay particular attention to them. Also, we only pay attention if we have some idea of where to look. Hence, reflection can be understood as a mental faculty dealing with the products of sensation and perception.

Given that clinical supervision can be enhanced through reflective practices, it is necessary to provide some understanding of what reflective practices are and also what purposes they serve.

In nursing, reflection is often described as a structured means by which relevant practice knowledge may be identified, reviewed and made sense of either individually or in groups — just as in clinical supervision. Atkins and Murphy (1993) highlighted the need for individuals to be open-minded and motivated when reflecting, and outlined five main skills helpful for reflection. These are:

Self-awareness: *honestly asking how the individual affected and was affected by a situation.*
Description: *the ability to recognise, recollect and describe situations as well as feelings and emotions.*
Critical analysis:*challenging assumptions, exploring alternatives and asking the relevance of knowledge in specific situations.*
Synthesis: *the amalgamation of new and previous knowledge in the move towards a new perspective.*
Evaluation: *making value judgements involving the use of criteria and standards.*
(Atkins and Murphy, 1993, pp.1188–92)

Reflection can be seen as thinking about what we do and several authors have provided some definitions of this. Dewey (1933) states that reflection is:

An active, persistent and careful consideration of any belief or supposed form of knowledge in the light of the grounds that support it and the further conclusion to which it tends.

(Dewey, 1933, p.9)

This definition appears to be rather unclear and difficult to interpret. A more user-friendly explanation is given by Boud *et al* (1985). This states that reflection is:

A generic term for those intellectual and effective activities in which individuals engage to explore their experiences in order to lead to a new understanding and appreciation.

(Boud *et al*, 1985, p.19)

Here Boud *et al* draw our attention to the fact that reflection helps individuals to concentrate on their feelings and beliefs so that an understanding of actions can take place thus allowing individuals to achieve professional maturity and confidence.

Reid (1993) identifies reflection as:

A process of reviewing an experience of practice in order to describe, analyse, evaluate and so inform learning about practice.

(Reid, 1993, p.305)

Here reflection is viewed in a cyclic manner whereby actions are reviewed, analysed and evaluated in order to provide either an improvement in practice or knowledge to enhance the quality of care. Van Manen (1990) describes four kinds of reflection:

1 *Anticipatory:* thinking about possible actions, interventions and outcomes.
2 *Active:* maintaining and promoting an awareness of what one is doing.
3 *Mindful:* developing the capacity to be actively reflective and thoughtful.
4 *Re-collective:* considering the success of actions and interventions.

No brief résumé of reflection can go without a mention of the significant contribution that Schon (1983, 1987) has made to our understanding of reflection. Schon describes two kinds of reflection, namely reflection-in-action and reflection-on-action.

Reflection-in-action

Reflection-in-action is utilising issues such as past experiences, individual values, opinions and expectations 'on the spot'. It has a critical function in that the knowledge we have is questioned and, consequently, our actions may be restructured. Reflection-in-action could be classified as 'critically thinking on your feet'. The handling of situations which were previously dealt with automatically is now questioned: why are they handled that way, and what are the possible consequences?

Reflection-on-action

Reflection-on-action, according to Schon, takes place after the event and needs to be guided so that thinking and practice can be moved forward. This is what clinical supervision intends to do and, in order for this to be effective, a reflective conversation needs to occur (Ghaye, 2000, Ghaye and Lillyman, 2000).

A reflective conversation can show evidence of one or more of the five types of reflection-on-practice described by Ghaye *et al* (1996a). These are descriptive, perceptive, receptive, interactive and critical-type reflections.

Descriptive   is the individual's personal, comprehensive retrospective account of a situation.

Perceptive   contains explanations for the feelings of the individual.

Receptive   reflection-on-action provides a justification for practice and offers a link between the individual's thinking, feelings and practice and those of others.

Interactive   reflection shows a link between learning from reflection and future action. A rationale for action is given with the aim of moving practice forward.

Critical   reflection-on-practice challenges the status quo and examines the structures that serve to liberate or constrain practice. Without this it is often impossible to improve practice.

Some of the purposes of reflection

Reflection has many purposes. As Ghaye (1996) suggests, it:

- acts as a bridge from the tacit knowledge to the considered action, and from the practice world to the process of theory generation
- enhances quality of action as it allows individuals to talk about their practice and provide different methods of work which can be tried out
- increases individual and collective accountability
- allows the status quo to be challenged constructively and yet critically.

What are some of the understandings of clinical supervision?

Recommendations following the Allitt Inquiry (Clothier *et al*, 1994) highlighted the necessity for supervision for safe and accountable practice. Clinical supervision was thought to be a way of preventing such tragedy recurring in nursing by protecting standards and developing expert nursing care as identified in the Department of Health (1994) publication, 'Clinical Supervision for the Nursing and Health Visiting Professions'.

The document entitled *Post Registration Education and Practice* (UKCC, 1994) aimed to create a framework for standards of education and practice for post-registration nurses, midwives and health visitors. It highlighted the present need to develop supervision of practice whilst enhancing care and maintaining standards. It stated that: 'all nurses, midwives and health visitors must demonstrate that they have maintained and developed their professional knowledge and competence' (UKCC, 1994, p.4). The Department of Health (1993) document, *A Vision for the Future* (Target 10), also supported clinical supervision and it was seen as having an important impact on improving nursing practice and accountability.

Clinical supervision is not a mandatory requirement for nurses, but has been a statutory part of midwifery practice for some time. However, support networks have been available to practitioners on an ad hoc basis for years. Clinical supervision is seen as a more formal version of this. It can help nurses to develop theory and practice, and relate skills and knowledge. The UKCC (1996) *Position Statement on Clinical Supervision for Nursing and Health Visiting*, endorses the implementation of clinical supervision in order to maintain and improve standards in healthcare.

Many definitions of clinical supervision are espoused, some being more comprehensive and some more understandable than others. Most definitions emphasise the benefits of supervision and support similar key qualities of it.

> *Clinical supervision is a term used to describe a formal process of professional support and learning which enables individual practitioners to develop knowledge and competence, assume responsibility for their own practice and enhance consumer protection and the safety of care in complex situations. It is central to the process of learning and to the expansion of the scope of practice and should be seen as a means of encouraging self assessment as well as analytical and reflective skills.*
>
> (Department of Health, 1993, p.15)

Butterworth (1994) stated that clinical supervision is:

> *... an exchange between practising professionals to enable the development of professional skills.*
>
> (pp.32–34).

Castledine (1994) enriches the debate by suggesting that clinical supervision:

> *... means different things to different people. For example, to a nurse manager it means inspection and checking of a worker's performance by someone who is looking only for things that are done wrong.*
>
> (p.1135)

One of the clearest understandings of clinical supervision is that:

> *... it is a meeting between two or more people who have declared an interest in thinking again about an aspect of healthcare work. The work is presented and they collectively think about what was happening and why, what was done or said, and how it was handled. This would normally include a discussion of issues such as: could it have been handled better or differently, and if so, how?*
>
> (Wright, 1989)

The definition of clinical supervision within our own NHS Trust (Alexandra Healthcare NHS Trust Hospital, 1995a) is that:

> *Clinical supervision is a support network for professionals,*

by professionals, encompassing all aspects of nursing whilst maintaining professional standards and developing expertise. During the process of personal and professional reflection, guidance and support is given.

Some functions of clinical supervision

In the past, nursing has tended to rely on hands-on experience to develop individual expertise. However, such factors as expanded clinical practice, increased autonomy, and a greater degree of decision-making have combined to increase the need for effective and personally meaningful clinical supervision. In our experience clinical supervision, when effectively introduced and nurtured by the 'power-brokers' within the Trust, works extremely well for the practitioner. It can provide an opportunity to critically analyse situations and, in turn, can lead to improved practice and standards. Moreover, clinical supervision provides a forum for nurses to be supported by reflecting orally, or in written work (for example in learning journals) on their experiences. Implemented sensitively and appropriately this process may well help to improve staff morale and enhance the quality of care.

Clinical supervision can therefore be seen as a process which safeguards standards of patient care and advances nursing practice through reflection. We would wish to argue that its objectives might usefully be seen as follows:

- to provide support and guidance with issues related to the person and their professional practice
- to maintain and improve standards of care in the clinical area
- to enhance expertise
- to encourage learning through reflection
- to provide feedback on clinical practice
- to improve communication between professionals.

By reflecting on standards of practice and providing constructive feedback, practitioners' skills and professional values may well be enhanced and clarified. This may then have a positive impact on practice. Clinical supervision is an opportunity to clarify clinical 'realities' and this, in turn, can serve to empower nurses (Ghaye, 2000).

In working with our colleagues we have found that fruitful areas for discussion and reflection in the clinical supervision context may include:

- the analysis of critical incidents
- the review of workload
- a constructive critique of standards of care
- support of personal concerns.

It is necessary for professional practice nurses to work in a safe and accountable manner at all times. This can only be achieved by constantly improving and updating knowledge, skills and sensitivities and it requires training and education of which clinical supervision is an integral part. As Bishop (1994) states:

> *While clinical supervision can help nurses to achieve the best level of care possible, it cannot compensate for inadequate facilities, poor management, or for unmotivated staff. However, it can create a culture within which nurses can flourish, if they are willing to accept it, and if management are supportive.*

We suggest that the benefits of clinical supervision can be represented as follows:

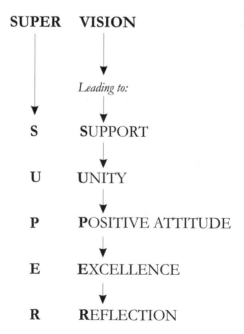

SUPER   VISION

Leading to:

S	SUPPORT
U	UNITY
P	POSITIVE ATTITUDE
E	EXCELLENCE
R	REFLECTION

In today's nursing profession, the rate of change is greater than ever before. These changes may either be welcomed or resisted. Clinical supervision provides a formalised mechanism for discussing issues and opportunities related to these changes.

Furthermore, by setting time aside to acknowledge best practice and discuss difficulties, clinical supervision offers a way to manage change more effectively. Clinical supervision is, therefore, a potential benefit to managers, staff, members of the multi-disciplinary team, the hospital and patients.

The UKCC (1996) *Position Statement on Clinical Supervision for Nursing and Health Visiting*

This:

> *endorses the establishment of clinical supervision in the interests of maintaining and improving standards of care in an often uncertain and rapidly changing health and social care environment. The UKCC commends this initiative to all practitioners, managers and those involved in negotiating contracts as an important part of strategies to promote high standards of nursing and health visiting care into the next century.*

(p.5)

Castledine (1994) suggests that as nurses have greater autonomy and accountability than ever before, support, advice and mentor/ preceptorship is required for them to develop to their full potential. Despite all the literature available about clinical supervision there is relatively little that suggests how it might be successfully implemented and, even more importantly, how it might be sustained in practice. A popular view suggests that strategies for implementation should be agreed locally (UKCC, 1996). Consideration of the aims, objectives, ground rules, framework for discussion and confidentiality need to be discussed. Together these form part of that important thing called 'culture'. We have learnt that if the Trust culture is unsupportive of clinical supervision then it is likely to struggle to take hold. These are complex issues on which we have only touched here; they are further elaborated upon throughout this book.

Effective clinical supervision through reflective practices

If reflection is to be of any use, the individual (or group) being supervised needs to be able to recount experiences honestly. A safe and supportive context needs to be created. For some the asking and responding to key questions helps in re-telling and re-experiencing. Some of the questions might be:

- What did I/we do?
- Why did I/we do it like this?
- How has it come to be this way?
- How can I/we improve it?
- What serves to inhibit or foster this intention?

Working towards improvement

Very busy emergency departments can leave nurses worrying about incidents that happen when there is little or no time to discuss or reveal their feelings at the time. They may be concerned about their own or other people's actions. The introduction of clinical supervision should go some way to enabling nurses to understand their own feelings, for as we know clinical action is influenced by both how we feel and think. Reflection can reveal to us how self and collective understandings can, if harnessed and subjected to critique, lead to our at least conceptualising what improvements in practice might be. This cannot be done if clinical supervision is seen as something quite separate from reflective practices, or is undertaken with a poor understanding of the potential for transformation promised by reflection (Johns and Freshwater, 1998).

Fish and Twinn (1997) described reflection-on-practice as being at the very heart of quality clinical supervision. They acknowledged that reflection seeks to heighten the critical awareness and critical consciousness of nurses in order to enhance their ability to think independently and exercise wise, ethical and competent professional judgements.

Seeing reflection as central to effective clinical supervision means, by implication, that we have a professional commitment to strive to improve our thinking about practice — practice itself and/or the clinical context in which practice takes place. Thought about in this way, reflection becomes a set of principles and processes that enables us, individually or collectively, to move forward. It is about an improvement process, not a change one. Not all change is improvement. There will, of course, always be some resistance to embracing reflection for purposes such as this. The process of managing resistance of one form or another arguably becomes more manageable when broken down into four stages. These are:

1 Shock and resistance.
2 Confusion.
3 Integration.
4 Acceptance.

Although these stages over-simplify reality, the labels are nevertheless useful in helping us to understand a complicated process.

Shock and resistance

Shock and resistance is created by the desire to maintain the *status quo*, even though clinicians might not be entirely happy with it. It is easier to stay within a comfort zone. All staff are aware of the *Code of Professional Conduct* (UKCC, 1992) which states that:

> *... each registered nurse, midwife or health visitor is accountable for their practice and, in the exercise of their accountability, must acknowledge any limitations in their knowledge and competence, and assist professional colleagues in the context of their own knowledge, experience and sphere of responsibility, to develop their professional competence.*
>
> (p.2)

Traditionally nurses have been discouraged from dwelling on the psychological stresses arising from the job. Similarly, they have been encouraged to leave their personal lives at home. After years of practice, most nurses will have mastered the art of the stiff upper lip. Hence, no wonder there is a resistance to taking the lid off stored-up emotions. Some nurses resist clinical supervision because there is insufficient time available to really explore how they feel about their work. A few minutes here and there, a chat over a coffee or conversations in one's own time are not what clinical supervision should be about.

Confusion

Confusion, which is caused when our certainties are questioned, can represent the beginning of a process of acceptance where the possibility of alternative ways of approaching things becomes more apparent.

Integration

Integration is where staff begin to consider actively how new insights and opportunities might be 'taken on board' and used to move their practice forward. This is not an easy process; it is often an emotional as well as a cognitive one. It can be bumpy and take much longer than at first thought. Talking things through with 'critical friends' in the context of the reflective conversation is important here. This can help staff to 'work it out'; to be sure of the meaning and impact of what they are thinking about upon their practice. Conversations of this kind can also promote of a sense of self-worth.

Acceptance

Acceptance is where individuals and groups become increasingly comfortable with the idea and the consequences of doing things differently. Acceptance often involves a change in values and actions. Values affect what we do; they are the reasons why we do the things we do. Practice is values-in-action. An acceptance that improves practice in a particular way will almost always involve, at least, a reappraisal of existing values and an acceptance of the provisionality of them.

How can reflective practices through clinical supervision make an impact in a critical care setting?

We wanted to reflect the philosophy put forward in the *Mission Statement* of our Trust: 'The Trust will strive for excellence in providing safe, effective quality care' (Alexandra Healthcare NHS Trust Hospital, 1995b) as it applied in a critical care setting. We decided, therefore, to look specifically at the admission areas of both accident and emergency, together with the emergency assessment unit.

By definition, emergency admissions are acutely ill or injured people. They can arrive at an assessment unit or accident and emergency department as individuals or in large numbers. Often the heaviest workload will arrive over the shortest period of time. Stress can arise because of the need to respond to a patient's needs on an intuitive emotional and clinical level, quickly and effectively.

Arguably the nursing process has little to offer in emergency situations. Benner *et al* (1992) state that assessment, planning, intervention and evaluation are exposed as arbitrary stages that inadequately represent how practitioners make decisions. In practice these stages are not isolated but work in a dynamic and interactive way where assessment of what is and evaluation of what has been, happens at the same time as intervention. To work competently, safely and accountably we have to be able to reflect-in-action. Clinical supervision, informed by guided reflection, for staff in critical care settings might help them to come to terms with their own feelings and actions. It will help them to understand how far they can realistically live their values out in their practice, as well as making them more aware of what they know and need to know.

When considering a 'practice incident' with a supervisor, staff can reflect upon how they handled clinical and managerial issues. This also provides an opportunity to discuss policy and procedures in the light of current events, and to question the need for improvement. As all staff begin to accept clinical supervision and as their reflective skills develop, the learning gained from previous experiences can help them make more informed and justified decisions at stressful times.

Undertaking clinical supervision demands a high degree of commitment from staff at all levels. Such commitment will be both practical and philosophical. Practically, there has to be a willingness to spend time and effort; philosophically, there has to be a belief in the effectiveness and benefits of a supervisory system. All staff must be prepared to look critically at the quality of their own practice. Clinical supervision has the potential to be a powerful learning process. It is essential, therefore, that it is used with sensitivity and understanding. Clear boundaries and safeguards are needed to protect both supervisor and supervisee. Some kind of learning contract — or at least some ground rules — should be negotiated and agreed at the beginning of any supervisory session. For example, it is important that the extent and limitations of confidentiality are clarified and agreed. An understanding of what does and does not fall within the scope of clinical supervision must also be established. Frequency and length of meetings, record-keeping and other practical details should also be included. Such a contract should be for a fixed period of time and should be subject to review.

It would appear that promoting reflective practices through clinical supervision is the way forward if we wish to have thoughtful, accountable, safe practitioners. But introducing clinical supervision into a busy critical care area does pose some issues as highlighted by Marrow *et al* (1997). Time is the main constraint on the process of clinical supervision. Working around internal rotation, holidays and heavy demands of work, means that arranging supervision sessions is very difficult. We cannot stress enough the need to gain full support from Trust management if the Trust is serious about making clinical supervision a worthwhile and professional activity.

With regard to reflective practice, it can be viewed as navel gazing and some practitioners believe that this is a habit they employ naturally and in which they do not need guidance. Johns (1996) believes that some practitioners may struggle to use a reflective model of nursing because it challenges their commitment to therapeutic work. This may be uncomfortable. Other nurses may prefer to objectify both their patients and themselves as a way of avoiding the emotions of working with people. Also, we found that some staff find certain subjects too painful to voice and accordingly become less than open. When the supervisor gets too close to their true feelings they will often ask that they have a change of supervisor. Therefore, the role of supervisor must also include the promotion of trust and the raising of awareness within those being supervised.

In order to illustrate our own personal thinking, we decided to prepare one concept map each according to the process set out by Ghaye *et al* (1996b). Concept maps are a way of describing, on paper, what it is that we are thinking. They reflect some 'big ideas' or concepts and the links or relationships between them that we have in our minds. They are, then, 'mind maps' that we can use to help us to reflect on things. They can also act as catalysts for discussion, particularly if concept maps about the same set of ideas can be compared and explained through group discussion. We decided to try to explore the connections in our minds between clinical supervision and reflection. We spent some time discussing what we felt would constitute a limited number of key concepts associated with the area which would help to trigger the connections we had about them in our minds. In addition to 'clinical supervision' and 'reflection', we added 'values', 'theory', 'practice', 'safeguard standards' and 'critical analysis'. We created different maps — (see *Figures 5.1* to *5.3* on *pages 88* and 89). On all the maps, the interconnectedness of the key concepts is apparent.

Figure 5.1, on *page 88*, shows how important it is to label the lines between each concept. In this way, our thinking becomes more public and therefore open to scrutiny and inspection. As a group of three nurses discussing our work afterwards, we felt that *Figure 5.1* contained some important messages. Firstly, the multiple and important roles of reflection are drawn in. Secondly, we felt that the interactive relationship between practice and theory was highly significant. Theory was not separated from practice. Thirdly, the association between reflection and clinical supervision through the cognitive processes of critical analysis raised much discussion. This was a particularly valuable feature of the concept map, as much has been written recently about the importance of nurturing critical thinking in healthcare and its role in the development of clinical judgement and effective healthcare interventions (Chenoweth, 1998; O'Neill and Dluhy, 1997; Bethune and Jackling, 1997).

Figure 5.2, on *page 89*, represents the same ideas in a very different way. We were particularly interested to talk through three big messages that it contained. Firstly, we talked about how it reflected the view that one of the purposes of 'clinical supervision with reflection' was to 'change' practice and theory. Secondly, we discussed the idea portrayed on the left side of the map; that our values make up our 'theories' of nursing and that these 'theories' in turn guide our practice. Finally, we used the map to explore the complementary notion, on the right side of the map, that our values give our practice its shape, form and purpose, and that our practice is evidence of our 'theories-in-use'.

We decided that *Figure 5.3*, on *page 89*, showed us that reflection-in-action and clinical supervision (that is, reflection-on-action) both supported a single aim, namely to maintain and safeguard standards of patient care in clinical settings. Critical analysis of practice fuelled these reflections. Secondly, critical analysis also needed to be applied to our professional values, theory and practice. This was seen as essential in developing competence, safe practice and accountability.

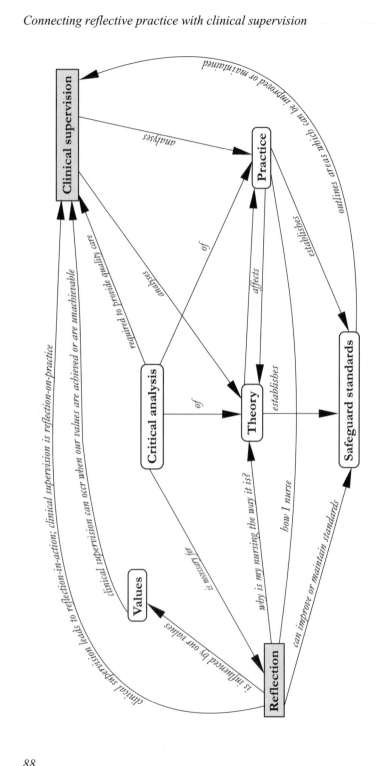

Figure 5.1 A labelled-line concept map showing some links between reflection, clinical supervision and related ideas

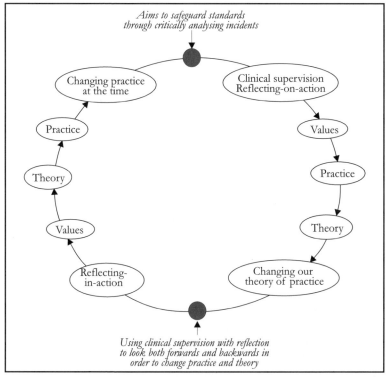

Figure 5.2: A labelled line concept map showing some links between reflection, clinical supervision and related ideas

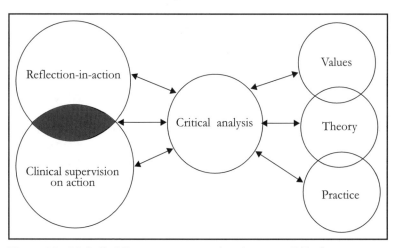

Figure 5.3: A labelled-line concept map showing some links between reflection, clinical supervision and related ideas

Some final thoughts

Both reflection-in-action and reflection-on-action through clinical supervision are seen as an entitlement of every practitioner in order to safeguard and to promote the interests of individual patients. Effective clinical supervision through reflection also serves to improve professional knowledge and competence as stipulated in Clauses 1 and 3 of the *Code of Professional Conduct* (UKCC, 1992). For successful implementation, management support and a 'culture' ready and sensitive to its introduction, is required.

By reflecting on the concept maps on *pages 88* and *89*, we began to appreciate more richly and holistically that our practice was value and theory laden, and that values and theories were both interlinked and crucial in supporting the delivery of high standards. We then also began to appreciate that if clinical supervision was to be a learning experience for those involved, then it might be prudent to consider a range of ways in which learning through reflection could be facilitated. We believe that concept-mapping activities could have an important place in fostering learning from experience. It is now very clear to us that it is not possible to consider effective clinical supervision without its resting on a firm understanding and appreciation of reflective practices. If clinical supervision is viewed as a learning experience then it needs to be a reflective process. If it is viewed merely as technical problem-solving and fire-fighting, and does not involve a consideration of goals and values, means and ends, then it is something else and something less. Clinical supervision viewed in this way reduces healthcare professionals to technicians and enslaves us once more in what Schon (1983) called 'technical rationality'. If clinical supervision is not richly permeated by the principles and processes of reflective practices, how can we make claim to be anything other than 'technicians'? If we do not embrace reflection we will never have the opportunity to question the values that underpin our practice and make us the kind of healthcare professionals that we claim to be. If clinical supervision is not a reflective process then we will never question the contexts in which we work and how the structures that influence all that we do serve to liberate or oppress, marginalise or empower us.

References

Alexandra Healthcare NHS Trust Hospital (1995a) *A Definition of Clinical Supervision.* Alexandra Healthcare NHS Trust Hospital

Alexandra Healthcare NHS Trust Hospital (1995b) *Mission Statement.* Alexandra Healthcare NHS Trust Hospital

Atkins C, Murphy K (1993) Reflection: a review of the literature. *J Adv Nurs* **18**: 1188–92

Bethune E, Jackling N (1997) Critical thinking skills: The role of prior experience. *J Adv Nurs* **26**: 1005–12

Bishop V (1994) Clinical Supervision for an Accountable Profession. *Nursing Times.***90**(39): 35–7

Boud D, Keogh R, Walker D (1985) *Reflection: Turning Experience into Learning.* Kogan Page, London

Boud D, Walker D (1991) *Experiencing and Learning: Reflection at Work.* Deakin University Press, Geelong

Benner P, Tanner C, Chelsea C (1992) From beginning to expert gaining a differential clinical world in a critical care setting. *Advances in Nursing Science* **14**(3): 13–28

Butterworth T (1994) Preparing to take on Clinical Supervision. *Nursing Standard* **8**(52): 32–4

Cameron B, Mitchell A (1993) Reflective peer journals: developing authentic nurses. *J Adv Nurs* **18**:290–7

Castledine G (1994) What is Clinical Supervision? *Br J Nursing* **13**(21): 1135

Chenoweth L (1998) Facilitating the process of critical thinking for nursing. *Nurse Education Today.* **18**: 281–92

Clothier C, McDonald C, Shaw D (1994) *Independent inquiry into deaths and injuries on the children's ward at Grantham and Kestever General Hospital during the period Feb to April 1991.* (Allitt Inquiry) HMSO, London

De Bono E (1979) *Wordpower.* Penguin, Harmondsworth

Department of Health (1993) *A Vision for the Future.* HMSO, London

Department of Health (1994) Clinical Supervision for the Nursing and Health Visiting Professions. *Chief Nursing Officer's Professional Letter.* **94**(5) DoH, London

Dewey J (1933) *How we Think.* Henrey Regney, Chicago

Fish D, Twinn S (1997) *Quality Clinical Supervision in the Health Care Professions.* Butterworth-Heinemann, London

Ghaye T, ed. (1996) *Reflection and Action for Healthcare Professionals: A Reader.* Pentaxion Press, Newcastle upon Tyne

Ghaye T, Cuthbert S, Danai K, Dennis D (1996a) *An Introduction to Learning through Critical Reflective Practice, Self-supported Learning Experiences for Healthcare Professionals.* Pentaxion Press, Newcastle-upon Tyne

Ghaye T, Cuthbert S, Danai K, Dennis D (1996b) *Professional Values: Being a Professional, Self-supported Learning Experiences for Healthcare Professionals.* Pentaxion Press, Newcastle-upon Tyne

Ghaye T (2000) Empowerment through reflection: Is this a case of the Emperor's new clothes? in Ghaye T, Gillespie D, Lillyman S, eds (2000) *Empowerment Through Reflection: The narratives of healthcare professionals.* Quay Books, Mark Allen Publishing, Salisbury

Ghaye T, Lillyman S (2000) *Reflection: Principles and practice for healthcare professionals.* Quay Books, Mark Allen Publishing, Salisbury

Johns C (1996) The benefits of a reflective model of nursing. *Nursing Times* **92**(27): 44

Johns C, Freshwater D, eds (1998) *Transforming Nursing through Reflective Practice.* Blackwell Science, Oxford

Marrow C *et al* (1997) Promoting reflective practice through structured clinical supervision. *J Nurs Man* **5**:77–82

O'Neill E, Dluhy N (1997) A longitudinal framework for fostering critical thinking and diagnostic reasoning. *J Adv Nurs* **26**: 825–32

Popper K (1965) *Conjectures and Refutations.* Routledge and Keegan, London

Reid B (1993) 'But we're Doing it Already!' Exploring a response to the concept of reflective practice in order to improve its facilitation. *Nurse Education Today* **13**: 305–9

Schon D (1983) *The Reflective Practitioner: How practitioners Think in Action.* Basic Books, New York

Schon D (1987) *Educating the Reflective Practitioner.* Jossey Bass, San Francisco

UKCC (1992) *Code of Professional Conduct for the Nurse, Midwife and Health Visitor.* UKCC, London

UKCC (1994) *Post Registration Education and Practice.* UKCC, London

UKCC (1996) *Position Statement on Clinical Supervision for Nursing and Health Visiting.* UKCC, London

Van Manen M (1990) *The Tact of Teaching: The meaning of pedagogical thoughtfulness.* University of New York Press, New York

Wright, H (1989) *Groupwork: Perspectives and Practice.* Scutari Press, London

6

An alternative training approach in clinical supervision

John Cutcliffe

Some current issues in clinical supervision training

Clinical supervision continues to be one of the central nursing issues within the National Health Service (NHS) (Cutcliffe and Burns, 1997). The National Health Service Management Executive (NHS ME, 1993), the UKCC (1995) and the King's Fund (1995) all advocated the implementation and use of clinical supervision for all practitioners. Recent literature reiterated this point of view with Bond and Holland (1998) asserting the need for all practitioners in all clinical areas to receive supervision. It is reasonable to say that many nursing researchers, academic nursing departments and self-governing NHS Trusts have indeed responded to this need, and clinical supervision is increasingly being incorporated into nursing strategies within faculties, departments and directorates (Farrington, 1995).

In the light of the continued attention that clinical supervision in nursing receives, it is worth examining briefly how the need for this practice originated. The argument in favour of formalised support mechanisms for nurses in the form of clinical supervision was pioneered by Professor Tony Butterworth in the early 1990s (Butterworth, 1991; 1992). Additionally, reported work from other professions was gradually beginning to influence thinking in nursing (Butterworth *et al*, 1996), and supervision models from counselling and psychotherapy were starting to be incorporated into nursing practice (Proctor, 1986; Hawkins and Shohet, 1989). Subsequent to these developments, according to Bishop (1994a), the significant factors to emerge from the UKCC *Code of Professional Conduct* (1992a) and *The Scope of Professional Practice* (UKCC, 1992b), are the individual's increased accountability combined with the demise of traditional support systems, which make clinical supervision essential. Furthermore, the findings of the Allit enquiry (Clothier *et al*, 1994) emphasised the need for safe and accountable practice.

Clinical supervision within nursing was then endorsed by the Chief Nursing Officer of the Department of Health who considers it to be fundamental to safeguarding standards, the development of expertise and the delivery of quality care (DoH, 1994).

Alleged benefits

Ultimately, the fundamental purpose of clinical supervision is improvement in client care, and this can be regarded as the principal benefit. At the same time, it is also alleged that clinical supervision brings about benefits for clinicians. These alleged benefits are:

- increased feelings of support and feelings of personal well-being (Butterworth *et al*, 1996)
- increased knowledge and awareness of possible solutions to clinical problems (Dudley and Butterworth, 1994)
- increased confidence, decreased incidence of emotional strain and burnout (Halberg and Norberg, 1993)
- higher staff morale and satisfaction leading to a decrease in staff sickness/absence, and increased staff satisfaction (Butterworth *et al*, 1996
- increased participation in reflective practice (Hawkins and Shohet, 1989)
- increased self-awareness (Cutcliffe and Epling, 1997)

Current attempts to research these alleged benefits centre around the three components suggested by Proctor (1986), these being normative (that is, organisational, professional ethics and quality control), restorative (support for staff) and formative (education and development). Indeed, initial findings from Butterworth *et al*'s (1997) multi-site study, which explored several questions of clinical supervision, provided some evidence to suggest that receiving clinical supervision does benefit the recipient, in particular in the realms of reducing emotional exhaustion and depersonalisation. Furthermore, qualitative and anecdotal evidence exists suggesting that clinical supervision can improve client care (Paunonen, 1991; Booth, 1992; Timpson, 1996; Cutcliffe and Burns, 1997).

The introduction of clinical supervision in practice

As indicated above, many of the self-governing NHS Trusts have already begun to implement clinical supervision. Evidence for this implementation is found in the anecdotal accounts that proliferate in current nursing literature (Hallberg and Norberg, 1993; Barton-Wright, 1994; Coleman, 1995; Everitt *et al*, 1996; Fisher, 1996; Fowler, 1996a; Fowler, 1996b; McGibbon, 1996; Morcom and Hughes, 1996; Wilkin *et al*, 1997; Wright *et al*, 1997). Examination of these papers indicates that there is no one singular method of implementation. However, it is clear that the one commonality all these attempts share is that any training provided is centred around equipping and enabling individuals to become supervisors, not supervisees. Whilst this approach has benefits, it also has major drawbacks which warrant further consideration.

The drawbacks of training nurses to be supervisors

Clinical supervision is a specific skill. Whilst a number of the interpersonal skills utilised in supervision may be transferable from nurse or counselling training, clinical supervision goes far beyond basic interpersonal abilities and has its own unique set of skills. Consequently, there is a need for specific clinical supervision training. Yet there is no standardised minimum quality and no widely accepted definition of what constitutes clinical supervision training. Within Butterworth *et al*'s (1997, p.17) multi-site study it is reported that the respondent sites had offered a wide variety of training opportunities:

> *Courses and training ranged from 6.5 days to 1 day, most commonly 2–3 days.*

This cross-sectional view of clinical supervision training reflects the experience of the author. His contact with self-governing NHS Trusts, higher education institutions and those individuals who offer clinical supervision training privately, indicated a wide range of practices and desired outcomes, all under the general umbrella of clinical supervision. The diversity in the quality of the training may well have a detrimental effect on the quality of supervision provided. Cutcliffe (1997) argued for the need to examine if a correlation exists between the level or intensity of supervision training given and the extent of positive outcomes in terms of benefits to clients and clinicians. The author suggests that it is not unreasonable to postulate that if a nurse receives insufficient or inappropriate training in clinical supervision, then the quality of clinical supervision they provide is unlikely to be capable of producing measured change implying either improvement in the supervisees' mental well-being, or improvements in the care they provide.

However, enabling every potential supervisor to attend quality supervision training presents many logistical problems. High-quality training is likely to be relatively lengthy and expensive when compared with the other options, such as in-service training. Smith (1995) reported that a director of patient care and nursing estimated that it would cost around one hundred thousand pounds to implement clinical supervision based on the calculation that each nurse in her hospital would receive two hours of supervision per month. It is unclear whether or not these calculations take into account the cost of training the nurses to become supervisors, this could therefore be considered a conservative estimate. Admittedly, a counter argument exists that suggests that one hundred thousand pounds is not really very much, representing as it does the cost of employing one NHS Trust chief executive for a year (Smith, 1995). This problem is further exacerbated if Regional Health Authorities do not provide additional funding to pay either for the training or for additional nurses to ensure that the wards are adequately staffed whilst the training occurs. Furthermore, as we operate in a climate where economics play an increasingly important role in determining the strategic planning of Trusts, the realistic and reasonable position of these organisations is to say that they cannot afford to release large numbers of staff to undertake extensive, intensive and expensive training courses, especially if there is a paucity of empirical data that conclusively supports the assertion that clinical supervision will benefit both clients and staff.

Problems with implementing clinical supervision in nursing

In addition to the absence of a plausible economic option for Trusts, the culture of the NHS does not yet have the infrastructure necessary for the widespread uptake of clinical supervision. Some of the problems relate to the limited understanding of clinical supervision practice. How can managers be expected to facilitate the equipping of nurses to the necessary extent if the nurses themselves do not possess this understanding? Fowler (1996a, p.382) supported this argument, suggesting:

> *Nursing and health visiting does not, as yet, have a culture of clinical supervision for qualified nurses. If we have little or no experience of being supervised ourselves, how do we clinically supervise others?*

Smith (1995) stated that feedback from participants at the NHSE conference on clinical supervision upheld this very viewpoint. Conference participants argued that a cultural shift was needed in order to progress the clinical supervision agenda into the whole organisation and that, crucially, clinical supervision may be needed but it also has to be wanted. Bishop's (1994b) survey of nurses' attitudes towards clinical supervision indicated that only 0.2 per cent of the *Nursing Times'* estimated readership actually responded to the questionnaire.Whilst workload pressure and slow circulation rates may account for some of this very low response rate, a distinct lack of interest in clinical supervision must surely also be considered as a reason (Bishop, 1994b). Furthermore, less than half of this sample (46 per cent) had clinical supervision up and running. Therefore, it is reasonable to suggest that there are many nurses who do not want clinical supervision at this time. Such resistance has many reasons for its existence, including:

- a tradition and culture that discourages the public expression of emotion
- the perception of clinical supervision as yet another management monitoring tool
- the perception of supervision as a form of personal therapy
- a continuing lack of clarity regarding the purpose of supervision
- resistance itself is an unavoidable component of the process of change (Wilkin *et al*, 1997).

The author argues that, when considering the resistance to clinical supervision, there is a crucial point that needs attention, and that is the apparent continuing lack of clarity regarding the purpose of supervision in nursing. An examination of the current literature highlights two separate perspectives on the purpose of clinical supervision. One view appears to conceptualise clinical supervision as an opportunity for a more experienced nurse to monitor, educate and support a less experienced nurse in how they carry out practical skills. This would create the need for all supervisors to be more 'expert' in the particular speciality of nursing than their supervisees. Alternatively, there is another view that appears to conceptualise clinical supervision as an opportunity to help and support nurses to reflect on their dilemmas, difficulties and successes, and to explore how they reacted to, solved or achieved them. This view puts supervision forward as a forum for considering the personal, inter-personal and practical aspects of care in order to develop and maintain nurses who are skilled and reflective practitioners. Such a situation creates the necessity for supervisors to be effective in supporting nurses in self-monitoring, identifying difficulties in practice and finding the proper place to make good the deficit — and not necessarily to be more expert themselves in the particular nursing speciality. This pivotal difference is seldom spelled out in the nursing literature and, consequently, it is not surprising that a sense of confusion exists for many nurses. Confusion concerning the very purpose of clinical supervision appears to create a resistance, and nurses seem to be unsure about what they are entering into.

The author has stated previously that despite this resistance some Trusts and educational institutions have made real progress in the implementation of supervision, and such endeavours should be applauded. If these efforts are then combined with systematic review and action research that produces evidence supporting the link between receiving supervision and improved client care/positive outcomes for staff, then resistance may begin to decline. However, such change will take time and may be somewhat parochial. The author argues that whilst implementation should be encouraged, what is needed is a radical shift in the emphasis of training staff in the practice of clinical supervision. An alternative approach is needed — one that features training nurses to be supervisees — and it is this alternative approach that warrants further examination.

Alternative approaches to training

It is interesting to note that feedback from the NHSE conference on clinical supervision (Smith, 1995) argued that training was necessary but that creating special courses should be avoided. The first point of this statement certainly supports the author's argument that clinical supervision is a specific skill, yet the second point perhaps casts some doubt on this issue. Surely, if clinical supervision is a specific skill, does that not denote the need for specific training? Perhaps there is an argument here for providing a standardised training; a training that would be available to all nurses. If all nurses are to become familiar with the practice of clinical supervision, and if clinical supervision should become a part of every nurse's career (McLoughlin, 1995), then there may be merit in examining how other common training requirements for nurses have been met.

All qualified nurses share a commonality in that they undertake a certain period of training before qualifying. Given that there is an identified need for some form of training for clinical supervision and that all nurses have this common experience prior to becoming qualified, *the logical solution to this problem is to incorporate clinical supervision training into pre-registration nurse training.* However, the crucial difference of this training would be that student nurses would be trained to be supervisees and not supervisors. This has many advantages and these will be discussed later, however, it also addresses the problems identified above, in that this form of clinical supervision training reduces the need for lengthy and costly post-registration clinical supervision training. The author is not suggesting that by training all student nurses to be supervisees the need for post-registration training is removed, *but rather that a common foundation, used in nurse training, would establish the framework on which future supervision experience can be built.* It would set in place, for the future, cohorts of new practitioners who could use supervision well, even if the supervisors were limited in their knowledge and application of supervision. Additionally, it would provide fertile foundations to act as the blocks of material needed for training supervisors. Consequently, new supervisors could build on their training and experience as 'good' supervisees, rather than starting from scratch.

Perhaps what this method of training would do most effectively would be to change the climate from the bottom upwards. Whilst it would not meet the training needs of those nurses who are already qualified, it would reduce the amount of time which future nurses would spend in post-registration supervision training, since they would already possess a basic understanding and experience of clinical supervision. As a result, post-registration training in clinical supervision would be shorter, and so save a great deal of money. Additionally, the supervisee training would be relatively straight-forward to standardise so that each nurse education centre provided at least the same minimum quality of training, thus addressing the problem of the wide diversity evident in current supervision training.

Training student nurses to be supervisees

Advantages of supervisee training

In addition to the substantial reduction in training costs and the possible standardisation of supervisee training, this approach brings further advantages. These are listed below and then discussed in greater detail. They are:

- the creation of greater equality and intentionality in the working alliance
- the increased awareness and understanding that supervision is something for the supervisee
- the sharing and agreeing of values, ground rules, terms and aims between the supervisee/supervisor and the organisation
- a sense of comradeship between peers; a greater sense of team cohesion; a counteraction to a culture of divide-and-rule
- the development of basic interpersonal skills (for example reflecting on practice, choosing issues, asking for and using help appropriately) in a less personally threatening forum.

The creation of greater equality and intentionality in the working alliance

Clinicians' resistance to supervision includes justifiable concerns that it is yet another management monitoring tool (Wilkin *et al*, 1997) and that, consequently, the locus of control (Rotter, 1972) remains very much with the supervisor. Such a position can be further understood when a consideration of current training methods suggests that supervisees will be entering into the supervision with little (if any) idea of what to expect. The current training is aimed at enlightening nurses about how to supervise, not about how to be a supervisee. If students are well-equipped to become supervisees, they are placed in an empowered position. Their awareness and experience of the supervision process during their training could thus enable them to realise that they are not 'done unto' during supervision. There is more equity in the distribution of power. Indeed, Hawkins and Shohet (1989) suggested that evaluation within supervision is a two-way process where both parties have the opportunity to give and receive open, honest, constructive feedback. Inskipp and Proctor (1989) argued that there is a joint responsibility for the supervision and thus supervisees need to be active in seeking what is the right sort of supervision for themselves. If subsequent supervision should start to move away inadvertently from support, development, growth and education and become custodial, punitive, or disabling, the student's knowledge and experience of the process could then enable them to deal with this more effectively and seek help in bringing the supervision back within the defined boundaries. The intentionality is increased in that both supervisor and supervisee are aware of the reasons for their time together. Hawkins and Shohet (1989) pointed out that this intentionality helps supervisees to become more proactive in gaining the support they need. Thus, the supervision becomes truly a shared responsibility; a purposeful, deliberate, conscious act of support, education and development aimed at facilitating client care, and ceases to be an ambiguous and amorphous concept.

The increased awareness and understanding that supervision is something for the supervisee

Current introduction of clinical supervision may well be viewed by nurses as yet another imposition from the nursing hierarchies. If supervision is seen as serving the organisation rather than the client or the clinician, then it is understandable that resistance exists. In order for this resistance to be counteracted, nurses need to discover that clinical supervision is indeed primarily for themselves and their clients, not just something for the supervisor, and certainly not something primarily designed as a tool for the management of the organisation. By making supervisee training an integral component of nurse education, students would be acclimatised to the experience of supervision and encounter the benefits for themselves. This argument is supported by Bishop (1994b), who reported that 98 per cent of nurses who had previously participated in peer review expected to benefit from clinical supervision. There appears to be a phenomenon here whereby the experience of receiving quality clinical supervision rapidly removes any misconceptions, anxieties, and resistance. Fowler's study (1995, p.37) also corroborates this argument. He examined the perceptions of post-registration nursing students regarding the elements of good supervision, and suggested that a key finding from stage three was that:

> *... all students wanted to see evidence of supervisors putting themselves out and helping the student build on their knowledge base.*

Students who had experienced supervision felt it had been provided for themselves, and wished to see evidence of this in the behaviour of the supervisor. Whilst the sample size in this study (fifty students from two courses) represents only a fraction of the population of nursing students, it provides a valuable insight into the world of students. This increased awareness that exposure to supervision generates also addresses the issue raised in the first part of this paper: that of confusion concerning the purpose of clinical supervision and the subsequent resistance this confusion creates.

Ritter *et al* (1996) described a model of clinical supervision which was provided to undergraduate general nursing students who undertook clinical placements on psychiatric wards. The model incorporates Schon's (1987) work on reflective practice and coaching whereby each student is helped to identify and articulate their experience on their own behalf and in their own way, in other words it makes attempts to be supervisee led. Ritter *et al* (1996, p.155) stated:

> ... *the model of clinical supervision enables students to choose to demonstrate their understanding by turning up to the supervision with something quite different from what the supervisor asked for.*

The students who became self-directed in their supervision appear to have grasped that the supervision is actually for themselves. Whilst this model appears to be a move towards training supervisees as it has an element of being supervisee led, it is still driven and guided by the supervisor. It is only when the supervisee has some understanding of the process and structure of the supervision that it becomes more completely supervisee led and, consequently, that supervisees are able to acknowledge that the supervision is indeed for themselves. How much more would the students benefit from this supervision if they began their placement already equipped with an understanding of what clinical supervision is for and what it is to be a supervisee.

The sharing and agreeing of values, ground rules, terms and aims between the supervisee/supervisor and the organisation

If all student nurses were provided with the same supervisee training, this could then create a commonality in the perception of the roles and tasks of supervision, and how these can be distinguished from other similar roles and tasks. White (1996) submitted that the term 'clinical supervision' has yet to be universally distinguished by practitioners from preceptorship, individual performance review or personal therapy. He goes on to suggest that debriefing and provision of the opportunity to reflect on clinical incidents was universally welcomed by the students in his study. Therefore, whilst students may have been unclear of the values, ground rules, and terms of supervision prior to receiving supervision, the actual participation in the practice of supervision produced a joint ownership. Once more, the value of providing students with experience of being a supervisee during nurse training is illustrated. Supervisee training exposes the student to the process of negotiating ground rules, and the need for this explicit contracting is identified by Proctor (1988), who stated:

> *If supervision is to become and remain a co-operative experience which allows real rather than token accountability, a clear — even tough, working arrangement needs to be negotiated.*

In addition, an awareness of the aims of supervision is increased. The student can begin to appreciate how supervision contributes to client, clinician and organisational need as a result of the increased self-awareness that clinical supervision can bring (Cutcliffe and Epling, 1997). When given supervisee training, the students can start to appreciate their need for development and, importantly, the personal responsibility they have for their own development. The student can begin to see how clinical supervision affects the way they deliver care and, consequently, the quality of care they provide. Similarly, such improvements in care will probably be part of the organisation's philosophy and/or strategy and thus both student and managers can see how the aims of supervision also contribute to meeting organisational need.

A sense of comradeship between peers; a greater sense of team cohesion; a counteraction to a culture of divide-and-rule

It is reasonable to suggest that traditionally nurses have been encouraged to contain their emotions and keep a lid on things. Many anecdotes exist of nurses crying in the sluice room having just dealt with yet another emotionally traumatic interpersonal situation. Such habitual repression can only bring about a sense of isolation and inadequacy, especially if the nurse believes that her peers regard her as someone who cannot cope because she weeps or lets off steam. Faugier (1992, p.27) also pointed out that nursing has a system loaded against the development of continued learning, fuelled by 'the threat of losing position or face before junior or untrained members of staff'.

For continuing learning to emerge from reflective practice, it is necessary for a culture of safety and honesty to be developed systematically. Supervisee training could then begin to eradicate debilitating and restrictive attitudes. What better way to begin to change the culture than by introducing students to the practice of reflection — of being open; of being able to recognise and express the impact of emotionally charged experiences, all of which are encouraged within well set-up clinical supervision? The increase in self-awareness that is brought about by participating in supervision (Faugier, 1992; Cutcliffe and Epling, 1997) enables trainees and nurses to realise when they need to express emotion and obtain support and, very importantly, that such processes are healthy — furthermore, that such processes are an integral component of each nurse's professional life. It also encourages them to realise that 'mistakes' are usually opportunities rather than marks of failure. The appreciation of a shared experience; of participating in a common, widespread phenomenon, creates a collective sense of cohesion. Furthermore, the support he or she experiences in supervision enables the nurse to think, 'I am cared for by these people; I am not on my own; I belong to this team.'

The development of basic interpersonal skills (for example reflecting on practice, choosing issues, asking for and using help appropriately) in a less personally threatening forum

Training students to be supervisees creates an environment where students need to enter into reflective practice, self-examination of learning needs, and practising being assertive. Yet all this can occur in a forum where there is no punitive presence, because the under-pinning essence of supervision is support. Students who experience this support in supervisee training, and conceptualise that in order to support one needs to listen actively and empathise (Burnard, 1989), arguably become more capable of providing such effective support. Butterworth (1992) hypothesised that students who are trained in a learning environment that encourages active listening, empathy and support will, in turn, become qualified nurses who foster similar therapeutic exchanges between other nurses and patients. This argument is supported by Cassedy and Cutcliffe (1998), who reasoned that students need to experience in counselling training the kind of empathy, genuineness and respect for their own personhood that the author wants them to be offering to clients. This entire training ideology of nurturing qualities is captured by Connor (1994, p.37) who stated:

> *Qualities are not developed by just practising skills or writing essays. They develop through the sum total of the learning experience and they are more likely to develop if there is intentionality in the learning process through ongoing structural experiences of reflection, reviewing and objective setting.*

A suggested structure of supervisee training in nurse education

One possible structure for this training is as follows.

Year one: Teaching provided on the theory of supervision, including:

- definitions of supervision and delineation from related concepts
- models of supervision
- a historical overview of its inception
- how the processes of reflection and self-examination are interwoven with supervision
- roles of supervisees/supervisors
- ground rules and boundaries
- the process of contracting
- giving and receiving feedback
- ethical issues in supervision.

Year two: Following early clinical placements, students would have a minimum of one hour per month of supervision using material they had recorded in their personal learning journals. The particular format of this supervision, (that is, one-to-one or group) would be determined partly by the human resources available and partly by the number of students attending each course. In addition to the benefits of receiving the supervision, at the end of each module, placement or term, feedback could be given to the student on their use of supervision. How evident was it that the student participated in the roles, responsibilities and expectations of a supervisee? Had they taken responsibility for the actions, reflections and learnings? Did they appreciate their own needs for support?

Following this, the student would complete a case study which would include details of participation in and the influence of supervision. The student would need to illustrate their active participation in supervision and show how this influenced their client care and personal/professional development. This would include a written piece of work, but could also include audio or videotaped sessions of their practice.

Problems with training students to be supervisees

This alternative approach to training is not without its problems. One argument against the idea centres around the issue that this process would have to be experiential, with students using material from their own clinical practice as a source of learning (Schon, 1984). However, since students would be at an early stage of their training, they may have insufficient critical incidents or clinical material to bring to the clinical supervision sessions. Clinical supervision, the argument goes, would not be relevant until the students had some clinical practice. Another problem might be that students at this early stage in nurse training are too inexperienced to have an awareness of what they do not know or what they need to know. Individuals would only gain an awareness of their deficits once they had faced clinical situations and found themselves lacking. There is also the issue that trained supervisees could conceivably produce feelings of anxiety and disempowerment in their subsequent supervisors. These new practitioners would be able to use supervision well and would not require such highly trained supervisors. However, being faced with a supervisee who knows more about the process of supervision may be unnerving. Supervisors may well be anxious that they are unable to deal with the issues the supervisee raises.

In reply to these arguments there is a case for first training students in the theory of supervision and then exposing them to the process, in the same way that students are taught the theory of interpersonal communication skills prior to these skills being utilised in a clinical environment. Therefore, the experiential component of this training would only commence after students had been on a clinical placement. As students accrued more experience, they would access more material that could be brought into the supervision session. The theory would already equip them with reasons why the processes that occur in supervision are necessary. The possible anxieties and feelings of disempowerment for a new supervisor are not exclusive to those individuals providing supervision to trained supervisees. The same feelings could well be present for any supervisor, as Hawkins and Shohet (1989, p.33) declared:

> *suddenly becoming, or being asked to be a supervisor can be both exhilarating and daunting.*

Additionally, if supervisors were equipped with information about the supervisee training, it could both inform and challenge their existing supervision practice.

A further problem may well occur in incorporating this training into an already cramped pre-registration nurse training curriculum. Whilst the author acknowledges this issue, he still feels the need to construct the argument for including training to become a supervisee at this early stage in each nurse's training. The specific infrastructure of nurse training curricula can be debated widely, and the argument this chapter puts forward can be included in those debates.

Evaluating supervisee training in nurse education

Butterworth *et al* (1996) showed that initial attempts to evaluate supervision centre around the three components suggested by Proctor (1986), these being normative (that is, organisational and quality control), restorative (support for staff) and formative (education and development), and that these provide a format for this evaluation (Butterworth *et al*, 1997). It would be logical for evaluation of supervisee training to follow a similar format. However, the author feels that evaluation in the normative category needs to be refined to ensure that the distinction between the supervisors' and supervisees' responsibility for overall normative development is clarified. This category needs to reflect very clearly their shared responsibility for learning, the internalising of professional ethics and standards of practice, and their shared responsibility for learning and developing competent practice. Crucially, comparisons would have to be made between a control group of students who receive no supervisee training and a group of students who do receive supervision training, measured in terms of Butterworth's multi-centre study.

Normative

Quantitative research into this component would centre on audit data concerned with rates of student sickness/absence and student satisfaction levels. In particular, do students find they are more satisfied with their training when it includes supervisee training? Qualitative data could include supervisee preparation. Additionally, in their case study (see above) students would be required to cite an instance where supervision has helped them with an issue of evaluating good practice or making an ethical decision, thus addressing the shared normative responsibility in supervision.

Restorative

Quantitative research into this component would centre around the measurement of the stress levels of students, a coping-levels questionnaire, and burn-out inventories. In particular, how supported and listened to do students feel on a course that provides supervisee training? How does being on a clinical placement and receiving supervision training compare to being on a placement that does not have this training? That is, does the training make it easier for the student to meet other educational criteria? Qualitative data would include the identifying of what being supported and listened to felt like on a course providing supervision training. For example, how did the training for supervision increase the students' confidence, well-being and creativity in a way that contributed to their meeting other educational and practice criteria?

Formative

Research into this area would centre around the evaluation of observed performance, for example in the form of audiotape records, videotape records, or observations of clinical practice. This method of evaluation has already been used on Thorn training courses. It could also include the case study assignment which would provide such qualitative evidence of the benefits of receiving supervisee training as comparisons between students' own experiences of clinical problems and how these were addressed. Also in the case study, trainees would be expected to include particular incidences of how supervision experiences had affected subsequent understanding and practice.

Conclusion

The practice of clinical supervision is considered by the chief officer of the Department of Health to be fundamental to the safeguarding of standards, to the development of expertise and to the delivery of quality care, and it is therefore reasonable to say that it is here to stay. It allegedly brings significant benefits to both clients and clinicians, and recent research has produced both quantitative and qualitative evidence to support this argument. Already, many Trusts have made attempts to introduce the widespread implementation of clinical supervision, with most of these developments being concerned with equipping clinicians to be supervisors and not supervisees. This presents several logistical and financial problems, and currently neither the infrastructure nor the culture is in place throughout nursing that would facilitate a widespread and effective uptake of clinical supervision. However, one alternative method of tackling this problem would be to include supervisee training within the CFP component of diploma nurse education and within the first two years of undergraduate nurse education. Training student nurses to be supervisees has several alleged advantages. These are:

- a substantial reduction in training costs and time
- a possible standardisation of training
- the creation of greater equality and intentionality in the working alliance
- the increased awareness and understanding in students that supervision is something for them
- the sharing of values, ground rules, terms and aims between the supervisee/supervisor and the organisation
- a sense of comradeship between peers in a culture that is often described as having an ethos of divide-and-rule, and a greater sense of team cohesion
- the development of basic interpersonal skills (for example, reflecting on practice, choosing issues, asking for and using help appropriately) in a less personally threatening forum.

An educational model would include both the theoretical and the experiential components, with the theory preceding the experience and thus addressing some of the arguments raised against supervisee training. Evaluation of this training would be carried out using a format similar to that used by Butterworth *et al* (1997) in evaluating the impact of receiving supervision. Finally, the concept of supervisee training is supported by Butterworth (1992, p.12), who states that:

> *Introduction to a process of clinical supervision should begin in professional training and education, and continue thereafter as an integral part of professional development.*

References

Barton-Wright P (1994) Clinical supervision and primary nursing. *Br J Nurs* **3**(1): 23–30

Bishop V (1994a) Developmental support for an accountable profession. *Nurs Times* **90**(11): 392–4

Bishop V (1994b) Clinical Supervision Questionnaire. *Nurs Times* **90**(48): 40–2

Bond M, Holland S (1998) *Skills of Clinical Supervision for Nurses.* Open University Press, Milton Keynes

Booth K (1992) Providing Support and Reducing Stress: a review of the literature. in Butterworth CA, Faugier J, eds, *Clinical Supervision and Mentorship in Nursing.*Chapman Hall, London

Burnard P (1989) The role of the mentor. *J District Nurs* **8**(3): 8–17

Butterworth T (1991) Setting our professional house in order. in Salvage J, ed. *Working for Change in Primary Health Care.* King's Fund Centre, London

Butterworth T (1992) Clinical supervision as an emerging idea in nursing. in Butterworth T, Faugier J, eds, *Clinical Supervision and Mentorship in Nursing.* Chapman Hall, London

Butterworth T, Bishop V, Carson J (1996) First steps towards evaluating clinical supervision in nursing and health visiting: I. Theory, policy and practice development. A review. *J Clin Nurs* **5**:127–32

Butterworth T, Carson J, White E *et al* (1997) *It is good to talk. Clinical supervision and mentorship. An evaluation study in England and Scotland.* The School of Nursing, Midwifery and Health Visiting, University of Manchester

Cassedy P, Cutcliffe JR (1998) Empathy, Students and the Problems of Genuineness. *Ment Health Practice* **1**(9): 28–33

Clothier C, MacDonald C, Shaw D (1994) *Independent inquiry into deaths and injuries on the children's ward at Grantham and Kesteven General Hospital during the period February to April 1991 (Allit Inquiry).* HMSO, London

Coleman M (1995) Using workshops to implement supervision. *Nurs Standard* **9**(50): 27–9

Connor M (1994) *Training the Counsellor: an integrative model.* Routledge, London

Cutcliffe JR (1997) Evaluating the success of Clinical Supervision. *Br J Nurs* **6**(13): 725

Cutcliffe JR, Burns J (1997) Personal, Professional and Practice Development using Clinical Supervision: Case Vignettes from Psychiatric Nursing. *J Psychiatr Ment Health Nurs* (accepted for publication: July 1997)

Cutcliffe JR, Epling M (1997) An Exploration of the use of John Heron's Confronting Interventions in Clinical Supervision: Case Studies from Practice. *Psychiatr Care* **4**(4): 174–5, 178–80

Department of Health (1994) CNO Letter 94(5) *Clinical Supervision for the Nursing and Health Visiting Professions.* HMSO, London

Dudley M, Butterworth T (1994) The Cost and some Benefits of Clinical Supervision: An initial exploration. *Int J Psychiatr Nurs Res* **1** (2): 34–40

Everitt J, Bradshaw T, Butterworth T (1996) Stress and clinical supervision in mental health care. *Nurs Times* **92**(10): 34–5

Farrington A (1995) Clinical Supervision: UKCC must be more proactive. *Br J Nurs* **5**(12): 716

Faugier J (1992) The Supervisory relationship. In Butterworth T, Faugier J, eds, *Clinical Supervision and Mentorship in Nursing.* Chapman Hall, London

Fisher M (1996) Using reflective practice in clinical supervision. *Professional Nurse* **11**(7): 443–4

Fowler J (1995) Nurses' perceptions of the elements of good supervision. *Nurs Times* **91**(22): 33–7

Fowler J (1996a) Clinical Supervision: What do you do after saying hello? *Br J Nurs* **5**(6): 382–5

Fowler J (1996b) How to use models of clinical supervision in practice. *Nurs Standard* **10**(29): 42–7

Hallberg IR, Norberg A (1993) Strain among nurses and their emotional reactions during 1 year of systematic clinical supervision combined with the implementation of individualised care in dementia nursing. *J Adv Nurs* **18**(1800–75)

Hawkins P, Shohet R (1989) *Supervision in the Helping Professions.* Open University Press, Milton Keynes

Inskipp F, Proctor B (1989) *Skills for supervisees and skills for supervisors.* (audiotapes) Alexia Publications, E.Sussex

King's Fund (1995) *Clinical Supervision: an executive summary.* King's Fund, London.

McLoughlin C (1995) *Clinical Supervision for Nursing and Health Visiting.* UKCC, London

McGibbon G (1996) Clinical supervision for expanded practice in ENT. *Professional Nurse* **12**(2): 100–2

Morcom C, Hughes R (1996) How can clinical supervision become a real vision for the future? *J Psychiatr Ment Health Nurs* **3**: 117–24.

NHS Management Executive (1993) *A Vision for the Future.* HMSO, London

Paunonen N (1991) Changes initiated by a nursing supervision programme: an analysis based on log-linear models. *J Adv Nurs* **16**: 982–6

Proctor B (1986) Supervision: A co-operative exercise in accountability. in Marken M, Payne M, eds, *Enabling and Ensuring.* National Youth Bureau and Council for Education and Training in Youth and Community Work, Leicester

Proctor B (1988) *Supervision: a working alliance.* (videotape training manual) Alexia Publications, E.Sussex

Ritter S, Norman IJ, Rentoul L, *et al* (1996) A model of clinical supervision for nurses undertaking short placements in mental health care settings. *J Clin Nurs* **5**: 149–58

Rotter JB (1972) *Applications of social learning theory of personality.* Holt, Rinehart and Winston, New York

Schon D (1983) *The Reflective Practitioner.* Basic Books, New York

Schon DA (1987) *Educating the reflective practitioner: Towards a new design for teaching and learning in the profession.* Basic Books Incorporated, New York

Smith JP (1995) Clinical Supervision: Conference by the NHSE. *J Adv Nurs* **21**(5): 1029–31

Timpson J (1996) Clinical supervision: a plea for 'pit head time' in cancer nursing. *Eur J Cancer Care* **5**: 43–52

United Kingdom Central Council for Nursing, Midwifery and Health Visiting (1992a) *Code of Professional Conduct for the Nurse, Midwife and Health Visitor.* UKCC, London

United Kingdom Central Council for Nursing, Midwifery and Health Visiting (1992b) *The Scope of Professional Practice.* UKCC, London

United Kingdom Central Council for Nursing, Midwifery and Health Visiting (1995) *Proposed Position Statement on Clinical Supervision for Nursing and Health Visiting.* UKCC, London

Wilkin P, Bowers L, Monk J (1997) Clinical Supervision: Managing the Resistance. *Nurs Times* **93**(8): 48–9

White E (1996) Clinical Supervision and Project 2000: The identification of some substantive issues. *Nurs Times Research* **1**(2): 102–11

Wright S, Elliot M, Scholfield H (1997) A Networking approach to clinical supervision. *Nurs Standard* **11**(18): 39–41

Index

A

A First Class Service: Quality in the New NHS, DoH, 1998 xiii, xv, 66, 72
A Vision for the Future, DoH, 1993 19, 22, 23, 42, 77
accountability 77, 87, 103, 112
  collective 77
  in nursing practice xv, 23, 24, 77, 78, 81, 83, 87, 93, 103
  individual 77, 83, 93
  of practitioners 80, 81, 83, 85, 86
  professional 56
accountable
  practice xv, 23, 24, 77, 78, 81, 83, 87, 93, 103
  practitioner 25
  profession 16, 91, 110
action 91
  options for 63, 67
  planning 48
  research viii, 43, 71, 72, 98
  resulting from reflection xvi, 8, 56, 76, 77, 82, 84
  thinking in 72, 92
actions 82, 84, 106
  awareness 39
  clinical xvii, 49, 59
  determined by values xvi
  improved xvii, 65, 77
  questioning 31
  reflection on 52, 57, 58, 59, 60, 66, 75, 76, 85
advocate
  for the patient 1, 55

aims
  of reflection 76
  of supervision 33–34, 74, 81, 87, 101, 103, 110
  of training 8, 12, 48, 100
autonomous practice 24
autonomy 48, 50, 51
  in nursing 24, 79
  of nurses 24, 81
awareness (*see also:* self-awareness) 33, 86
  gained from training 100, 101, 103, 106, 109
  of work pressures 11–12
  resulting from supervision/ reflection 35, 37, 40, 75, 82, 86, 94, 102
  seminars 45
awareness-raising 7, 8, 25, 29, 35

B

beliefs 68, 69
  communicating 41
  debilitating 60, 104
  put into practice 39
  questioned by supervision vii, 15, 19, 24, 30, 36, 39, 75
benefits
  of clinical supervision xvi, 3, 4, 6, 7, 8, 12, 13, 27, 78, 80, 85, 94, 109, 111
    for staff 5, 28, 29, 30, 45, 81, 94, 96, 101, 109
    for patients 5, 28, 29, 81, 94, 96, 109

benefits *cont.*
   of clinical supervision *cont.*
      for practice 29, 30
      personal 21
   of reflection 92
   of training 7, 96, 101, 102,
      106, 109
blame culture 29, 32
boundaries
   in clinical supervision 23, 85,
      101, 105
   organisational 23
   professional 38

C

care 24, 38, 71, 72, 80, 84, 98
   for staff 27, 32, 38
   improvements in 8, 37, 45,
      59, 66, 73, 75, 77, 79, 81,
      94, 96, 98, 103
   in supervision 2, 23, 38, 104
   nursing 17, 19, 40, 77, 81
   patient 24, 28, 29, 34, 35, 40,
      45, 66, 87, 94, 98, 101, 106
   patient-centred xvii, xviii
   Peplau's model of 32, 35, 38,
      40, 41
   quality of xv, 19, 23, 59, 66,
      75, 79, 94, 103, 109
   safety of 23, 24, 78
caring 40
   philosophy 23
   practice 66, 68
   values 24, 33, 39, 47, 49,
      61–62, 68, 70
   work 64
challenge
   commitment 86
   constructive 47, 64, 68, 70
   of clinical supervision 6, 35,
      39, 107

challenging
   practice 23, 24, 46, 47, 59,
      64, 68, 70, 73
   questions 31, 62
   the status quo xvi, 10–11, 76,
      77
   through reflection 64
   values and beliefs 19
client care 106
   facilitating 101
   improving 94, 98
clinical
   actions xvii, 49, 59, 82
   conversation
      creative 55–72
      reflective 59, 60–68, 70
      structure in 67
   effectiveness xvi, 66
   environment 2, 50, 73, 107
      pressures in 10, 12
      influence of 49
      culture of 49, 50
      disempowering 51
   governance vii, xv, 66
   judgement 87
   practice 29, 32, 46, 79, 106,
      109
   problems 94, 109
   safety 24
   support 27
colleague-centred care xv–xviii
commitment 20, 33
   and work pressures 12
   professional 51, 82
   shared 64
   to clinical supervision 12, 26,
      48, 85
   to learning through clinical
      supervision 59, 66
   to reflective practice 31, 64,
      66
   to therapeutic work 86

committed action 59
communication
   between professionals 79
communication skills 47, 53,
   107
   and reflective conversation
      63
competence 24, 72, 77, 87
   developing 23
   improving through clinical
      supervision 27, 78, 83, 88
   in supervision 58
   of practitioners 77, 78, 83
   professional 77, 83, 88
compromise 27, 65
   between time and supervision
      9, 12
compulsory
   clinical supervision 27
concept map 20–22, 25, 30–32,
   36, 37, 39, 41, 42, 86–87, 88,
   89, 90
   as a learning tool 86
confidence 25, 27
   and clinical supervision 27,
      38, 39, 94
   and empowerment 39
   and reflection 75
   and training 108
   breach of 25
confidentiality
   in supervision 15, 25, 47, 48,
      58, 81, 85
constraints 24, 40
   of time 5, 6, 7–9, 10, 11, 12,
      13, 26, 29, 34, 36, 48, 49,
      50, 81, 82, 83, 85, 86, 99
construction/reconstruction
   in reflection xvii, 57, 60, 64,
      65, 71
context
   historical 39, 60

context *cont.*
   of clinical supervision/
      reflection 52, 65, 66, 82
   of professional practice 20,
      57, 64, 65, 66, 83, 88
control
   and clinical supervision xv,
      25, 29, 32, 100
   by management 25, 51, 100
   of nurses 25, 29, 32, 66, 100
   personal xvii, 65, 66
conversational analysis 62
coping
   responses 51
   with change 19, 31
   with difficult situations 31,
      32, 104
cost-effectiveness
   of clinical supervision 6
creative
   clinical conversations 55
   experience in clinical
      supervision 47, 59, 63, 70
   patient care 24
   reflection 59, 60, 61, 64
   space 63
credibility
   and clinical supervision 5, 6,
      27
critical
   analysis 4, 13, 21, 36, 74, 76,
      79, 80, 85, 87, 91, 92
   awareness 82
   conversations 20, 42, 43
   distance 62
   friend 20, 84
   reflection 24, 43, 59, 64, 66,
      71, 76, 77, 91
   relationships 21
cultural changes 32, 34, 97, 104
culture 109, 110
   NHS 34, 96

culture *cont.*
  of blame 29, 32
  of clinical supervision 97
  of divide-and-rule 100, 104,
    110
  of reflection 22–23
  of the workplace xvi, 26, 32,
    34, 40, 42, 49, 50, 51, 80,
    81, 88, 97, 104, 110

D

debilitating beliefs 60, 104
decision-making 6
  and autonomy 50
  and practice development 67
  of practitioners 79, 85, 108
deconstructing 1
  incidents 36
definitions
  of clinical supervision 23,
    46, 78, 79, 91
  of reflection 74–75
development 87, 94, 100, 103,
  109, 110
  of clinical supervision 6, 28
  of knowledge 24
  personal 21, 28, 32, 35, 36,
    40, 103, 106, 111
  practice 67, 111
  professional vii, 10, 19, 21,
    34, 45, 73, 78, 94, 104, 106,
    110, 111
  vehicle 31
dialogue 42, 71
  of clinical supervision 55,
    62, 63
  reflective 20, 35, 55, 61, 63
dilemmas 42
  in implementing clinical
    supervision 2, 4–15
  in practice 98

dilemmas *cont.*
  of confidentiality 25
directorate business plan 6, 15,
  28
DoH
  1977 xv
  1993 19, 22, 23
  1994 19, 91, 94
  1998 xv

E

effective
  clinical pratice xvi, 26, 51,
    64, 66, 84, 85, 87, 88
  clinical supervision xvi, 33,
    35, 37, 49, 50, 60, 76, 79,
    82, 109
  management xi
  management of change 81
  practitioner 33, 53, 85
  reflection 75
  support 98, 105
  teams 52
efficiency 27, 50
empowerment
  of the individual xvii, 39, 41,
    65, 80
  through clinical supervision
    59, 80
  through reflection ii, xviii,
    33, 39, 41, 65, 71, 92
  through training 100
enabling process
  clinical supervision 47
  reflection 59
enlightenment
  through creative conversation
    65
environment 81
  clinical 12, 49, 50, 51, 73,
    107

environment *cont.*
  for clinical supervision 11, 35, 49
  training 104, 105
  working xvii, 11, 46, 50–52, 53
ethics
  in reflective conversation 60
  of enhancing quality care 59
  of reflective contract 58
  of supervision 105
  practice 64, 82, 108
  professional 94, 108
evaluation 74, 85
  in supervision 101, 106, 108
  of training 3, 7, 8, 9, 16, 48, 49–50, 107, 108, 109, 110
evidence
  in reflective conversations 76
  of benefits of clinical supervision 3, 5, 6, 27, 28, 67, 94, 98, 109
  of benefits of training 109
  of implementation of clinical supervision 95
  of practice 87
  of reflective conversations 62, 67, 68, 70
  of supervisor commitment 102
evidence-based medicine 6
evidence-based practice 27, 66–68
experience
  learning from 19, 24, 40, 47, 64, 65, 71, 75, 76, 79, 82, 85, 88, 91, 92, 104, 105, 107, 109
  of clinical supervision xvi, xvii, 2, 15, 20–21, 25, 34, 35, 36, 38, 46, 79, 88, 95

F

facilitation
  through clinical supervision 24, 52, 58, 65, 73, 91, 97, 101
  through reflective practice 37, 88
facilitator 2, 30, 47, 48, 50
feedback, in supervision 1, 17, 79, 101, 105
framework
  clinical supervision 4, 22, 24, 28, 34, 41, 47, 48, 65, 81, 92, 99
  for standards in education 77
  reflection 36, 47
framing and re-framing xv – xviii, 57
functions
  of clinical supervision xv, 40, 46, 79–81
  of reflection 76

G

group supervision xvi, xvii, 12, 13, 14, 16, 50, 66, 74, 82, 92, 106, 108
growth
  personal, through clinical supervision 26, 29, 32, 35, 36, 38, 40, 50, 51, 52, 101
guidance
  in supervision 3, 37, 79, 86

H

historical context
  personal/professional 39, 60
history of clinical supervision 93

holistic care xvii, xviii, 35, 38, 59

I

implementation of clinical
   supervision xv, xvi, 2, 4, 6, 8,
   11, 13, 14, 15, 16, 23, 24, 25,
   26, 28, 30, 32, 33, 41, 45–53,
   73, 78, 79, 81, 88, 93, 95, 96,
   98, 109, 111
improvement in practice xv,
   xvii, 8, 19, 23, 27, 36, 37, 40,
   45, 46, 56, 57, 59–60, 65, 66,
   67, 68, 73, 75, 76, 77, 78, 79,
   80, 81, 82–84, 85, 88, 94, 96,
   98, 103
innovation 32, 33, 41, 45, 51
in-service training 8–9, 10, 11,
   37, 48–49, 52, 95–98, 99,
   101–102
intentionality
   in supervision
      relationship100–101
   in the learning process 105

J

judgement
   clinical 87
   professional 36, 39, 41, 67,
      82

K

key concepts of clinical
   supervision 86–87
knowledge
   of/from clinical supervision
      xvi–xvii, 19, 23, 24, 30, 31,
      32, 39, 46, 47, 59–60, 73,
      74, 75, 76, 77, 78, 80, 88, 94

knowledge *cont.*
   professional 47, 56, 60, 77,
      83, 88

L

language (power of) 39, 55
learning
   contract 85
   from clinical practice 106
   journal (*see also:*
      record-keeping) 36, 41, 43,
      47, 71, 79, 106
   lifelong 15, 57, 66, 104
   needs 10, 30, 104
   shared responsibility 64, 101,
      108
   through clinical supervision
      19, 23, 24, 40, 47, 55, 59,
      62, 65, 66, 71, 78, 85, 88
   through reflective practice
      xvii, 75, 76, 79, 88, 91, 104,
      112
logistical problems
   of implementing clinical
      supervision 109
   of training provision 96

M

management 39
   attitudes to clinical
      supervision 5, 6, 9, 19, 23,
      25, 26, 28, 50, 51, 52, 80,
      86, 88, 93
   responsibilities 9
   tool (of clinical supervision)
      24, 26, 97, 100, 101
managers' attitudes to clinical
   supervision 5, 6, 9, 13, 14, 16,
   23, 24, 25, 26, 27, 28, 45, 46,
   50, 51, 78, 81, 97, 103

managing change 81
mandatory requirement
  for clinical supervision 26,
    27, 77
meaning
  of clinical supervision xv,
    xvii
  in reflective conversations
    46, 57, 58, 60, 63, 65, 68, 84
model
  of clinical supervision 2, 8,
    12, 38, 39, 40, 41, 58, 71,
    93, 102, 110, 112
  of patient-centred care xviii
  of supervisee training 110
  Peplau's 32, 35, 40
  reflective 86, 92
morale of staff 6, 29, 51, 79, 94
motivation
  for supporting clinical
    supervision 15, 23
  of staff 6, 25, 29

N

nursing
  and clinical supervision 16,
    17, 19, 93, 94, 96, 97, 109
  and reflection 40, 86
  care 17, 19, 40, 77, 81
  demands of 37
  model 35, 86
  practice xvii, 19, 20, 24, 25,
    47, 60, 68, 73, 74, 77, 79,
    81, 83, 87, 93, 97, 103, 104,
    108
  primary 32, 35
  profession 29, 32, 37, 38, 39,
    45, 68, 79, 81, 87, 97, 104
  strategies 93
  theories 68, 87, 93

O

one-to-one supervision 1, 12,
  73, 106
organisational
  attitudes to supervision 3, 6,
    9, 12, 13, 15, 23, 65, 96,
    101, 110
  boundaries 23
  influences 62, 94, 107
  philosophy/strategy 103
outcomes of clinical supervision
  5, 6, 16, 27, 58, 75, 95, 96, 98
ownership of clinical
  supervision 5, 103

P

patient
  advocate 1, 55
  benefits 3, 5, 28, 29, 45, 81,
    94, 96, 109
  care 23, 24, 28, 29, 34, 35,
    40, 45, 66, 79, 87, 94, 98,
    101, 106
  needs 26, 85, 88
  safety 25
  patient-centred care xvii,
    xviii
patterns of interest (in reflective
  conversations) 63
peers 35, 47, 100, 101, 104, 110
Peplau 38, 39, 41, 42, 43
  model 32, 35, 40
perceptions 50, 71, 74
  of clinical supervision 20,
    32, 97, 101–102, 103, 111
personal 48
  beliefs/feelings/values 15,
    32, 61
  control xvii, 65, 66
  experiences 32

personal *cont.*
  growth/development 16, 21,
    26, 28, 29, 32, 35, 36, 38,
    40, 50, 51, 52, 64, 101, 103,
    106
  history 39
  knowledge 47, 72
  learning journal 106
  motivation 23
  needs 32, 48, 80
  reflection 64, 73, 79
  viewpoint 20, 46, 76
  well-being 8, 94, 96, 108
political issues 52, 60, 63, 66,
  67
post-registration
  clinical supervision training
    99
  education and practice 77
power (*see also* empowerment)
  58
  bargaining 6
  brokers 79
  distribution 101
  of language 39, 55
  of reflection 34, 57, 65
practice
  accountable xv, 23, 24, 77,
    78, 81, 83, 87, 93, 103
  and theory/values 87, 88
  awareness of 30, 31, 32, 39,
    42, 47, 59, 62, 85, 109
  benefits to 29, 30
  challenging 23, 24, 46, 47,
    64, 68, 70, 73
  evidence-based 27, 66–68
  improving xv, xvii, 8, 19, 23,
    27, 36, 37, 40, 45, 46, 56,
    57, 59–60, 65, 66, 67, 68,
    73, 75, 76, 77, 78, 79, 80,
    81, 82–84, 85, 88, 94, 96,
    98, 103

practice *cont.*
  nursing xvii, 19, 20, 23, 24,
    25, 29, 47, 60, 68, 73, 74,
    77, 79, 81, 83, 87, 93, 97,
    103, 104, 108
  reflective xvii, 31, 34, 35, 37,
    38, 39, 40, 46, 47, 56, 57,
    64, 65, 66, 67, 73–92, 94,
    102, 104, 110, 112
  safe 26, 77, 93
  standards 73, 77, 109
practitioners 5, 6, 7, 16, 23, 24,
  25, 26, 28, 30, 33, 34, 43, 46,
  56, 58, 59, 60, 61, 65, 66, 67,
  72, 73, 77, 78, 79, 81, 85, 86,
  88, 92, 93, 98, 99, 103, 107,
  112
pre-registration nurse training
  99, 107
pressures
  clinical 10, 12
  time 34, 50
  work 6, 9, 10, 12, 29, 34, 50,
    51, 52, 97
problems 25, 29, 38, 57, 58, 59,
  60, 73, 88, 94, 99, 100
  implementing clinical
    supervision 4–15, 96–98,
    109
  of training 106–107, 109
professional ii, xvii, xviii, 2, 16,
  20, 23, 31, 38, 39, 43, 45, 46,
  48, 52, 55, 56, 58, 59, 60, 62,
  64, 65, 66, 71, 72, 73, 75, 78,
  79, 82, 83, 86, 88, 91, 92, 93,
  94, 104, 108, 110, 111, 112,
  113
  competence 77, 83, 88
  development vii, 10, 19, 21,
    39, 67, 73, 106, 110
  judgements 36, 39, 41, 67, 82
  knowledge 56, 77, 88

professional c*ont.*
  practice 51, 56, 60, 79, 80,
    93
  self-regulation vii, 15, 66
  support 23–24, 27, 46, 78, 79
  values 1, 8, 23, 42, 46, 59,
    61, 79, 87, 92
psychological stress 83
purpose
  of clinical supervision xvi, 4,
    8, 87, 94, 97, 98, 102
  of reflection 60, 74, 76–77,
    83

Q

quality
  care xv, 19, 23, 32–33, 40,
    59, 66, 75, 79, 84, 94, 103,
    109
  supervision 8, 9, 34, 42, 64,
    71, 82, 91, 95, 96, 101
  training 95, 96, 100
questions
  clinical supervision xvi–xvii,
    4, 5, 28, 31, 70
  reflection 61, 62, 63, 72
  training 8–10, 48
questioning
  approach 35, 39, 40, 59, 60,
    64, 70, 85
  practice/self 24, 27, 30, 31,
    61, 62, 76, 82, 88

R

reality 4, 6, 11, 57, 83
reconstructed practice 65
reconstruction xvii, 56, 57, 60,
  65, 71

record-keeping (*see also:*
  learning journal) 36, 47, 58,
  63, 67, 68, 86, 106, 109
reflection
  and clinical supervision 15,
    33, 34, 36, 37, 45, 56, 59,
    60–68, 79, 82, 85, 86, 87,
    88, 89, 90
  and practice 39, 46, 79, 87,
    105
  areas for discussion in 80
  definitions 74–75
  framework 36, 47
  purposes 76–77
  skills for 74
reflection-in-action/practice 34,
  56, 66, 75, 76, 85, 87, 88
reflection-on-action/practice 24,
  31, 34, 35, 52, 56, 59, 64, 66,
  75, 76, 82, 87, 88
reflective
  clinical conversation 59,
    60–68, 70
  contract 58
  conversations xvii, 4, 8,
    19–43, 46–48, 51, 55,
    56–58, 59, 60, 61, 62, 63,
    65, 67, 76, 84
  diaries 8, 27, 34
  model 86, 92
  posture 64
  practice(s) xvii, 8, 31, 34, 37,
    38, 39, 40, 56, 57, 61, 66,
    67, 73–92, 94, 102, 104
  practitioner 30, 56, 58, 66, 98
  process 35, 64, 88
  questions 62
  skills 19, 78, 85
reframing xvii, 57
relationship 4, 35
  challenging 21

relationship *cont.*
  clinical supervision 7, 8, 11,
    12, 14, 15, 16, 20, 21, 23,
    24, 34, 35, 39, 46, 48, 111
  interpersonal 50
  practice and theory 87
  staff and managers 6
  therapeutic 38, 40, 41
resistance
  to clinical supervision 9, 10,
    13, 25, 29, 97–98, 100, 101,
    102
  to reflection 83–84
responsibilities 9, 58, 106
responsibility 31, 32, 33, 108
  for practice 23, 24, 78
  individual 10, 23, 24, 78, 83,
    103, 106
  shared supervisor/supervisee
    64, 101, 108
roles 40, 55, 58
  model 26, 28
  of reflection 56, 60, 87
  of supervisee 106
  of supervision 103
  of supervisor 4, 7, 8, 9, 10,
    11, 14, 15, 25, 37, 68, 86
  professional 1

S

safe
  culture 104
  environment 35, 82
  practice xv, 23, 24, 26,
    33–34, 73, 77, 78, 79, 80,
    84, 85, 86, 87, 93, 94, 109
safety of care 23, 24, 78
scepticism about clinical
  supervision xiii, 20, 25
Schon xvii, xviii, 55, 56–59, 72,
  75, 76, 88, 92, 102, 106, 112

selection criteria 10
self 20, 51, 64, 65, 82
  sense of 20, 64, 65
self-assessment 19, 78
self-awareness 26, 27, 36, 37,
  40, 74, 94, 103, 104
  through supervision 103
self-critical 32
self-direction 37, 102
self-disclosure 48
self-examination 104, 105
self-monitoring 98
self-regeneration 66
self-regulation 15, 66
self-selection 10
self-sufficiency 50
self-worth 84
sharing
  commitment 64
  experience 35, 104
  reflections 41
  responsibility 64, 101, 103,
    108
  thoughts, ideas 37, 69
  values and beliefs 39, 100,
    110
  view of clinical supervision
    49
skills 47, 55, 60, 73, 74, 98, 105
  clinical supervision 30, 32,
    60, 95, 99
  interpersonal 47, 52, 95, 100,
    104, 107, 110
  practitioner's 24, 79
  supervisor's 7, 9
  professional 78, 80
  reflective 19, 62, 74, 78, 85
social structures 60
staff morale 94
standards of care/practice 74,
  81, 88, 108
  framework 77

standards of care/practice *cont.*
  improving 37, 73, 78, 79, 81
  maintaining 77, 79, 81
  protecting 77
  reflecting on 79, 80
  safeguarding 19, 73, 79, 87,
    94, 109
stress
  at work 35, 36, 40, 46, 51,
    83, 85
  in students 108
structures
  at work 88
  clinical supervision 23, 48,
    58, 67, 88, 96, 102
  practice 76
  reflection 74
  social 60
  supervision training
    105–106, 107, 109
supervisee 2, 3, 7,8, 23, 24, 28,
  30, 45, 47, 48, 51, 55, 61, 62,
  63, 64, 67, 68, 85, 95, 96, 98,
  100, 101, 102, 103, 106, 107
  training 98, 99, 100–109, 110
    advantages 100, 109
    evaluation 107–108
    structure 105–106
    theory/experience 110
supervisee/supervisor
  boundaries 85, 103
  commitment 64
  conversation 47, 51, 55, 62,
    63, 64, 67
  record 47
  relationship 24, 100, 101,
    103, 105, 108, 110
  responsibilities 64, 101, 108
  training for 45, 48–49
supervisor 2, 3, 4, 5, 7, 8, 9, 10,
  11, 12, 13, 14, 15, 16, 21, 23,
  24, 25, 27, 28, 29, 30, 35, 36

supervisor *cont.* 37, 39, 41, 45,
  46, 47, 48, 49, 51, 55, 62, 63,
  64, 67, 68, 70, 85, 86, 95, 96,
  98, 99, 100, 101, 102, 107,
  108, 109
support xv, 12, 15, 27, 29, 31,
  33, 34, 37, 39, 45, 51, 81, 104
  for clinical supervision 15,
    19, 23–24, 27
  for practice 19, 79
  for supervisors 10, 11
  from clinical supervision 3,
    15, 20, 25, 26, 30, 31, 35,
    38, 46, 50, 78, 7980, 87, 93,
    94, 96, 98, 101, 104, 105
  from context 52, 81, 82
  from NHS 19
  in training 12, 105, 108
  management, 5–6, 9, 13, 26,
    28, 50, 51, 52, 80, 86, 88
  networks 77, 79
  of DoH 77, 78
  professional 23–24, 27, 28,
    46, 78, 79
sustainability 48

T

team 8, 9, 11, 19, 21, 23, 27,
  28, 34, 52, 81, 104
  cohesion 100, 104, 110
  management 5
  spirit 51
teamwork 51
technical rationality 59, 88
*The New NHS: Modern,
  Dependable*, DoH, 1977 xv,
  xvii
The Reflective Practitioner,
  Basic Books, 1983 xviii, 56,
  72, 92, 112
theoretical knowledge 16, 19

theories 59, 60, 87, 88
  of nursing 68, 87, 93
theory 77, 86, 110
  and practice 87, 88
  change 33
  of supervision 105, 107
  Peplau's 38, 41
  professional 87
therapeutic relationship 38, 40, 41
time constraints/pressures 5, 6, 7–9, 10, 11, 12, 13, 26, 29, 34, 36, 48, 49, 50, 81, 82, 83, 85, 86, 99
'toolbox' mentality 60
tool
  clinical supervision 25, 97, 100, 101
  management 24, 26
Train the Trainer 8, 16, 30, 32, 42
training
  for supervision 5, 7, 8, 9, 10, 11, 12, 13, 14, 15, 16, 30, 32, 35, 37, 41, 45, 47, 48, 49, 52, 80, 93–113
  evaluation 3, 7, 8, 9, 16, 48, 49–50, 107, 108, 109, 110
  in-service 8–9, 10, 11, 37, 48–49, 52, 95–98, 99, 101–102
  post-registration 99
  pre-registration 99, 107
  problems 106–107, 109
  supervisee 98, 99, 100–109, 110

V

value
  for money 6
  judgements 74

value *cont.*
  of clinical supervision 1, 2, 6, 19, 27, 35, 42, 73,
values 7, 15, 19, 61, 68, 86, 87, 100, 103, 110
  base xvi, 23, 60, 62
  caring 24, 33, 39, 47, 49, 61, 62, 68, 70
  in practice xvii, 61, 62, 84, 85, 87, 88
  personal 24, 30, 35, 38, 39, 41, 61, 76, 84
  professional 1, 8, 23, 42, 46, 59, 61, 79, 87, 92
voice 55
  of patient 55
  of professional 55, 59
voluntary supervision 13
vulnerability
  in clinical supervision 25, 39, 41
  in reflection 31, 35

W

well-being
  from clinical supervision 8, 94, 96, 108
  and supervision training108
work pressures 6, 9, 10, 12, 29, 34, 50, 51, 52, 97